Praise for *American Nightingale*

"Through indefatigable research and a nearly obsessive quest to inhabit a great moment in time, Bob Welch achieves something rare among works of military history: He brings one person, a single extraordinary person, to vivid life upon the page. Read *American Nightingale*, and you'll never think of D-Day in the same way again."

—Hampton Sides, author of *Ghost Soldiers* and *Americana*

"Has the golden cast of *Saving Private Ryan*."

—Book Babes

"We have forgotten what they endured, and how much they hoped and fought and sacrificed, the young hearts who came to this country, and gave it their all. This book brings it back."

—Paul Greenberg, Pulitzer Prize–winning columnist

"Bravo, Bob Welch!"

—Doris Booth, Authorlink.com

"Welch's compelling biography of Lieutenant Frances Slanger illuminates the extraordinary courage and patriotism so emblematic of the valorous army nurses who served in World War II. His intriguing volume serves as a celebration of these unsung heroines. It represents a vaíuable contribution to the literature of nursing, women in combat, and military history."

—Mary T. Sarnecky, author, *A History of the U.S. Army Nurse Corps*

"[*American Nightingale*] may well start a sea change in public consciousness. No one who reads [it] will ever again assume that every military hero killed in action was, is, or will be male."

—Judith Bellafaire, chief historian of the Women In Military Service For America Memorial Foundation

"Reading *American Nightingale* is an intensely moving and unforgettable experience."

—Evelyn Benson, author of *As We See Ourselves: Jewish Women in Nursing*

AMERICAN NIGHTINGALE

THE STORY OF FRANCES SLANGER,
FORGOTTEN HEROINE OF NORMANDY

BOB WELCH

ATRIA BOOKS

NEW YORK   LONDON   TORONTO   SYDNEY

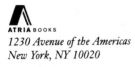
ATRIA BOOKS

1230 Avenue of the Americas
New York, NY 10020

ISBN: 978-0-7434-7759-8

First Atria Books trade paperback edition June 2005

10   9   8   7   6   5   4

ATRIA BOOKS is a trademark of Simon & Schuster, Inc.

Manufactured in the United States of America

For information regarding special discounts for bulk purchases,
please contact Simon & Schuster Special Sales at 1-800-456-6798
or business@simonandschuster.com

To the girl up the street,
Sally Jean

We leave you our deaths. Give them their meaning.

—ARCHIBALD MACLEISH

AUTHOR'S NOTE

In December 2000 a reader called me at *The Register-Guard* newspaper in Eugene, Oregon, where I'm a columnist. In an obscure book about Jewish women in the military, he had found a letter written to the *Stars and Stripes* newspaper by a World War II nurse, Frances Slanger. Nathan Fendrich, who teaches seminars about World War II and the Holocaust in area high schools, said the letter and the circumstances surrounding it had moved him like nothing else he'd read about the war. "She captures the American GI—the citizen soldier, the government issue—in a way I've never seen," he told me. "But what happened then . . . Well, you read lots of stories about guys falling on grenades, and that's heroic. This is a different kind of 'heroic.' "

Would I, Fendrich asked, consider writing a column about Slanger? Intrigued, I did so, pegging the piece to a World War II generation that's slipping from our national grasp. The response from the paper's 75,000-plus readers was warm, wide, and emotional, but one phone call stood out. It was from an eighty-two-year-old woman, Sallylou Cummings.

"My goodness," she said, "you've written about my friend Frances Slanger."

I was stunned. What were the chances of someone in Eugene, Oregon, having known a woman who had been born in Poland, had grown up in Boston, and had died in Europe nearly sixty years ago? I soon learned that Cummings, along with Slanger and sixteen other nurses, was part of the U.S. Army's Forty-fifth Field Hospital Unit. Wearing army fatigues and three-pound helmets, the women had splashed ashore at

Normandy four days after D-Day in June 1944. Along with another unit, they were the first U.S. nurses to step foot in France.

Cummings, who lives only ten minutes from my house, still had a copy of Slanger's letter as it appeared in *Stars and Stripes*. "We all remember the letter," she told me. She had photographs of the Forty-fifth's journey across France. She even had a handful of phone numbers of others in the unit whom she thought were still alive, though most names in her index-card file had lines drawn through them.

The story captivated me. For the next two years, I immersed myself in a search for Frances Slanger. The journey took me from Ellis Island to the location of Slanger's childhood row house in Boston; from the National Archives in Washington, D.C., to the homes, apartments, and assisted-living facilities of a handful of eighty-and-older people in six states; and, finally, from Utah Beach in France to a hillside cemetery far beyond.

Of the eighteen nurses in the Forty-fifth, I found only four still alive. Their memories—and the memories of six doctors and enlisted men I tracked down from the Forty-fifth—were the foundation on which this book is built. Also important was the considerable poetry and prose that Frances Slanger had written and kept in a personal "chapbook," along with inspirational writing by others.

As much as possible, I've tried to re-create Frances Slanger's story through her eyes and through the eyes of those who shared the journey with her. Dialogue and speeches in quote marks or indented form are either taken from written records or are reconstructions deemed accurate by those who were present at the time. Anecdotes are based on eyewitness reports, written accounts, or records. Some less significant contextual detail is based on recollections of those who encountered experiences similar to Frances's or on reasonable assumptions given time, place, and circumstances.

The Source Notes section at the book's end offers chapter-by-chapter substantiation for the incidents I've described. But my ultimate standard for credibility is having had the manuscript edited and approved by a nurse, a doctor, and a mess hall cook from the Forty-fifth Field Hospital Unit itself—those who were there.

Because of the passage of time and the deaths of so many witnesses, Frances Slanger's story can never be fully known. But based on what I was able to discover, this is the most accurate, complete, and realistic book I can write about her life and death.

BOB WELCH
Eugene, Oregon
May 2004

A RAINSTORM lashed the field hospital tent that had been home to Frances Slanger since the nurses had landed at Normandy so long ago. Artillery shells pounded in the distant darkness, by now so common that, like the rumble of the Boston Elevated Railway back home, Frances sloughed them off as the normal percussion of life. Not that such familiarity was helping her sleep; she had too much else on her mind. So she turned on a flashlight, found a pen, and wrote the following letter:

> It is 0200 and I have been lying awake for one hour, lis-
> tening to the steady, even breathing of the other three
> nurses in the tent. Thinking about some of the things we
> had discussed during the day. The rain is beating down
> on the tent with a torrential force. The wind is on a mad
> rampage and its main objective seems to be to lift the
> tent off its poles and fling it about our heads.
>
> The fire is burning low and just a few live coals are on
> the bottom. With the slow feeding of wood, and finally
> coal, a roaring fire is started. I couldn't help thinking
> how similar to a human being a fire is; if it is allowed to
> run down too low and if there is a spark of life left in it,
> it can be nursed back. . . . So can a human being. It is
> slow, it is gradual, it is done all the time in these Field
> Hospitals and other hospitals in the ETO.
>
> We had read several articles in different magazines
> and papers sent in by grateful GIs, praising the work of
> the nurses around the combat areas. Praising us—for

what? I climbed back into my cot. Lt. Bowler was the only one I had awakened. I whispered to her. Lt. Cox and Lt. Powers slept on. Fine nurses and great girls to live with . . . of course, like in all families, an occasional quarrel, but these were quickly forgotten.

I'm writing this by flashlight. In this light it looks something like a "dive." In the center of the tent are two poles, one part chimney, the other a plain tent pole. Kindling wood lies in disorderly confusion on the ground. We don't have a tarp on the ground. A French wine pitcher, filled with water, stands by. The GIs say we rough it. We in our little tent can't see it. True, we are set up in tents, sleep on cots and are subject to the temperament of the weather.

We wade ankle deep in mud. You have to lie in it. We are restricted to our immediate area, a cow pasture or hay field, but then, who is not restricted? We have a stove and coal. We even have a laundry line in the tent. Our GI drawers are at this moment doing the dance of the pants, what with the wind howling, the tent waving precariously, the rain beating down, the guns firing, and me with a flashlight, writing. It all adds up to a feeling of unrealness.

Sure, we rough it, but in comparison to the way you men are taking it, we can't complain, nor do we feel that bouquets are due us. But you, the men behind the guns, the men driving our tanks, flying our planes, sailing our ships, building bridges and to the men who pave the way and to the men who are left behind—it is to you we doff our helmets. To every GI wearing the American uniform, for you we have the greatest admiration and respect.

Yes, this time we are handing out the bouquets . . . but

after taking care of some of your buddies; seeing them when they are brought in bloody, dirty, with the earth, mud and grime, and most of them so tired. Somebody's brothers, somebody's fathers and somebody's sons. Seeing them gradually brought back to life, to consciousness and to see their lips separate into a grin when they first welcome you. Usually they kid, hurt as they are. It doesn't amaze us to hear one of them say, "How'ya, babe," or "Holy Mackerel, an American woman!" or most indiscreetly, "How about a kiss?"

These soldiers stay with us but a short time, from 10 days to possibly two weeks. We have learned a great deal about our American soldier, and the stuff he is made of. The wounded do not cry. Their buddies come first. The patience and determination they show, the courage and fortitude they have is sometimes awesome to behold. It is we who are proud to be here. Rough it? No. It is a privilege to be able to receive you, and a great distinction to see you open your eyes and with that swell American grin, say, "Hi-ya babe!"

The following night Frances Slanger was killed. She was the first American nurse to die in Europe after the D-Day landings at Normandy.

CHAPTER ONE

Die when I may, I want it said of me by those who knew me best, that I always plucked a thistle and planted a flower where I thought a flower would grow.

—ABRAHAM LINCOLN,
FOUND IN FRANCES SLANGER'S CHAPBOOK

The bow of the *William N. Pendleton*, a U.S. Merchant Marine freighter, sliced through the chop of the English Channel, cutting a wake soon lost in the trails of a hundred other ships. It was daybreak, Saturday, June 10, 1944, off France's Normandy coast.

From his lookout station on the bridge, a seaman scanned the waters with a slow, steady sweep of his binoculars. Beyond the swells that gently rocked the *Pendleton*, he saw the ships of the Allied Expeditionary Force—all sizes, all shapes—scattered across the Bay of the Seine. He saw the smoke-shrouded beach a few miles away, an occasional church spire jutting skyward beyond. And he saw the occasional floating corpse, a rag-doll remnant of the D-Day invasion four days before: some sailor who'd been on the destroyer USS *Corry* when it had hit a submerged German mine off Utah Beach. Or some GI in a life belt who'd been killed while landing at Omaha Beach and been sucked to sea by an outgoing tide.

Up top, deckhands and naval gun crews shouted to hear one another above the wind and drone of engines. The brackish gusts plastered the men's uniforms to their skin, clanged halyards, and whipped an American flag that splashed a rare touch of color from the after mast. Soon, muted sunlight burned through the smoke and mist that shrouded the Normandy shore. The *Pendleton* churned on toward the debarkation area. It was shortly before 6 A.M.

Like all of America's 2,710 Liberty ships, some of which were built by round-the-clock work crews in less than two weeks, the 441-foot *Pendleton* looked more like a cargo ship than a warship. Three masts jutted skyward, framing a squatty bridge amidships. Gaunt and devoid of portholes, she was painted a bleak gray with no lines, numbers, or anything else to distinguish her from other such craft. Guns were mounted on the fore and aft decks, small and obscured by the ship's sheer bulk. In 1941, when President Franklin Roosevelt had first been shown drawings of such a ship, he told Admiral Emory Scott Land that the Liberty appeared to be the kind of workhorse America needed to transport soldiers to battle. "She isn't much to look at though, is she?" he said. "A real ugly duckling."

Now, in the belly of one such duckling, 640 soldiers waited word to head for shore. They lay on canvas bunks that, stacked a claustrophobic four high, looked like trays in a baker's bread rack. They shuffled cards. Played craps. Talked. Argued. Boasted. Took drags on Lucky Strikes and Camels. Glanced at watches. Read one of the reduced-sized magazines published especially for troops. Some even whistled, presumably to remind themselves of how calm they were.

Ventilation ducts piped in fresh air, but it was quickly tainted by the stench of sweat, smoke, latrines, vomit, and the gaseous return of K-rations—not to mention the smell of some greasy substance that the soldiers' fatigues had been coated with to guard against the possibility of mustard gas. Spend a few days in the bowels of a Liberty ship, word had it, and you'd happily fight your way to shore.

In a narrow passageway on the troops' deck, a pug-nosed soldier stood outside a head, rocking lightly from foot to foot. "C'mon, c'mon," he said, hammering home his point with a knuckle rap on the door. "Speed it up, pal."

A moment later, the door swung open. The soldier froze. There in olive-green army fatigues stood a young woman with almost-blond hair. She was so stunningly out of context, so refreshingly unmale, so mind-numbingly gorgeous that the soldier momentarily forgot his bladder was about to burst like a grenade.

"Sorry," said 2d Lt. Sallylou Cummings. She smiled and tilted her head in a slight, if intentional, touch of flirtation. Then she limped past him, having torn ligaments in her left foot earlier that morning when a German glider bomb had jolted the ship.

Men weren't the only ones going ashore at Normandy. Nurses from the U.S. Army Nurse Corps were also aboard the *Pendleton*, including eighteen from the Forty-fifth Field Hospital Unit of which Cummings was part. Originally, the plan was for nurses to come ashore at least a week after D-Day, when their safety was more assured. But mounting casualties hastened their involvement. On D-Day alone, nearly 10,000 Allied soldiers had been killed or wounded in assaults on five beaches across a sixty-mile swath. Surgeons and medics were overwhelmed. Word came down from the Allied command center in England: Send the nurses to Normandy.

LYING ON HER port side bunk, Sallylou, a twenty-six-year-old Wisconsin girl, stuck a hand in one pouch to make sure she had her gas mask and another hand in a second pouch to make sure she had her makeup kit. Frankly, she was far more concerned about losing her makeup than her mask. She had joined the army because she didn't want to wind up working in a five-and-dime like her friends. And she had been so naive that she showed up for her first hike at Wisconsin's Camp McCoy wearing a pink dress and huarache sandals. She had no idea where she was headed, but wherever it was, she wanted to look good, which wasn't difficult for her.

She was five-feet-four inches tall, blue-eyed, and nicely curved. Despite her light brown hair, she had the look of a young Katharine Hepburn, which hadn't been lost on the guy waiting outside the head nor on other girl-starved military men, one of whom she had already fallen in love with. A soldier offered Sallylou a potato latke that had been sent from home. Though stale, it tasted better than some of the cold, unheated C-rations that some soldiers likened to wet cat food. "Thanks," she said.

Across the way, in a bottom bunk on the *Pendleton*'s starboard side, another nurse from the Forty-fifth lay on her stomach, gamely attempting to write a letter home amid the bob and pitch of the transport. She was thirty, short, and plump in a friendly sort of way. She had brown hair, brown eyes, a dark complexion, and a small mouth.

"Frances," said Sallylou, her voice raised to overcome the thrum of the engine and countless conversations and arguments, "do you ever stop writing?"

Frances Slanger hesitated, as if surprised she was being spoken to. "Lots to say after that air raid this morning," she said. "Bit more exciting than Fort Bragg, huh?"

Sallylou noticed how Frances's Boston accent had turned *fort* into *fawt*. "Anything's more exciting than Bragg," said Sallylou. "*Wisconsin* is more exciting than Bragg."

Frances laughed a little uneasily. Sallylou seldom talked to

Frances. She found the Boston nurse to be a quiet girl, a mysterious girl, though friendly enough when engaged in conversation—and the first Jew the Wisconsin nurse had ever met. Like most of the nurses in the Forty-fifth, Frances was from the Northeast, specifically from Boston's South End.

Sallylou Cummings was everything Frances Slanger was not. During training at Camp Ellis, Illinois, Cummings had been selected by an army photographer to pose for the *Chicago Tribune*. In a picture of her saluting the American flag, the count-me-in look on her face is so warm, earnest, and patriotic that it could have melted ice cream on Mom's apple pie. Meanwhile, Frances had, by accident, appeared in a *Boston Traveler* photograph that heralded the opening of a new cafeteria at Boston City Hospital. She is wearing thick glasses. Her self-conscious expression suggests a certain acceptance of her role in life as an "also-pictured" person.

And yet something about Frances Slanger intrigued people, among them Isadore "Tiny" Schwartz, a Jewish doctor who'd grown up in Quincy, Massachusetts, just south of Boston and was fast becoming Frances's closest friend. Even if some enlisted men considered Frances as cold as cod on ice and one captain called her "The Kike" behind her back, her uncommonness drew people to her.

Maybe it was the way she saw beyond herself, a woman whose good-naturedness inspired the inevitable clichés. "Pounding away at her typewriter with a heart of gold," Florence Sayer of Haverhill, Massachusetts, had written in Frances's "buddy book" after the two had shared a stint at Fort Devens near Boston. "She'd give you the shirt off her back."

Maybe it was the way she was so serious. She had a sense of humor, but she used humor like a lifeguard uses a life ring: with great effectiveness, but only in emergencies. Instead, she carried with her a certain world-on-her-shoulders heaviness, the kind of heaviness one might inherit from growing up in the squalid streets of World War I–torn Poland, which she did. And a heaviness one might absorb by clipping and pasting articles about how the Nazis despised the Jews, which she also did.

Maybe, as Forty-fifth Field Hospital Dr. John Bonzer realized, it was the way she saw more deeply than the rest, and took time to chronicle what she saw in words. Sometimes those words were hers and sometimes they were the words of philosophers and writers whose quotes she carefully cut out of magazines and pasted into a scrapbook-sized "chapbook" back home in Boston, but they spoke of the need to live an intentional life in pursuit of noble things. "Life is not to live merely, but to live well," reasoned the Roman philosopher Seneca in a quote Frances had saved. "There are some 'who lived without any design at all, and only pass in the world like straws on a river: they do not go; they are carried.' "

Even as a young girl, she had an almost extrasensory perception of life and her place in it. Frances was like a sailor who, so attuned to the sea, could tell the direction of the wind not only by looking at the telltales fluttering on the shrouds but by actually *feeling* that wind. Amid hundreds of thousands of troops pouring into France, then, she not only sensed the importance of what was happening, but believed she was keenly necessary to it all, as if it were part of some master plan that had begun that September day in 1920 when she'd arrived at Ellis Island.

Evil was threatening the world—the newspaper articles she clipped and saved said so—and must be stopped. And so when, like others on board, she had been handed her "order of the day," ostensibly written by Gen. Dwight Eisenhower himself to troops coming ashore at Normandy, she believed the man's words were written especially for her, 2d Lt. Frances Y. Slanger, U.S. Army Nurse Corps. "You are," he wrote, "about to embark upon the Great Crusade, toward which we have striven these many months. The eyes of the world are upon you. The hope and prayers of liberty-loving people everywhere march with you. . . .

"Your task will not be an easy one. Your enemy is well trained, well equipped and battle-hardened. He will fight savagely.

"But this is the year 1944! . . . The tide has turned! The free men of the world are marching together to Victory!

"I have full confidence in your courage, devotion to duty and skill in battle. We will accept nothing less than full victory!

"Good luck! And let us all beseech the blessing of Almighty God upon this great and noble undertaking."

Her going off to war, then, smacked of a certain personal destiny, some unseen force. She wanted to leave some sort of mark on the world. To make a difference. To *matter.* It was a lofty quest, given what the world had taught her the past three decades: that she didn't matter. Whether it was German soldiers in Poland who ransacked her family's flat, parents in Boston who reminded her that Jewish girls *don't* become nurses, or military bigwigs in Washington, D.C., who decided she was not fit for overseas duty, the message was always the same: you don't *go,* as the philosopher Seneca had said, you're *carried,* captive to the whims of the waters. But, in essence, her being on this ship—her going to war—marked a decision to start listening to herself.

The irony was that Frances Slanger hated war. In a poem she'd written, she pleaded with God to "Open the eyes of the aggressor nations so they will never forget the emptiness and futility of war/Open the eyes of their children and their children's children for generations to come." In an essay written in 1941, after Germany had attacked the Soviet Union, she wondered why "men have to go out to kill and be killed. Why?" She often prayed for peace.

Still, she also understood that, sometimes, the only way to stop a fire was to create a backfire, a short-term loss for a long-term gain. Death, yes, but not death without purpose. Death as a means of righting the wrongs of the world, which was what her hero, Gen. Douglas MacArthur, was trying to do in the South Pacific. "Dear God," she had written after marching in the Armistice Day parade in Dothan, Alabama, the previous November, "let our men rest in deep contentment with the knowledge that they have not died in vain. Let them see our hands clasped with all the people of the world."

In some respects, Frances Slanger was like the seventeen others in the Forty-fifth: just another adventure-starved young nurse who'd become an officer in the Army Nurse Corps, much to the dismay of some back home who believed such women were, at best, man-hungry hussies and, at worst, a threat to foul the entire American military machine. But in other respects, she was as different from the others as France's Normandy region was from its Alps.

FRANCES SLANGER's life was bracketed by war. She was fifteen months old when the ponies carrying the saber-wielding Cossacks first clomped through the cobblestone streets of Lødz, Poland, the horses' nostrils snorting steam in the brittle winter air. Grim-faced officers, clad in woolen greatcoats and topped with fur *papakha* hats, barked commands. Regiments of foot soldiers spread to posts at the city's outskirts. The officers' knee-high black boots dug into the horses' flanks and the animals bolted, some to the left, some to the right. Soon, the gossip birds on Piotrkow Street chattered with more dread than usual: Three months after the outbreak of World War I, the Russians, they'd heard, were bracing for battle with German soldiers who, even now, were rattling north on trains.

The burly city of Lødz (pronounced "Woodge") was a stepchild of the Russian Empire. It was a place where the textile factory whistles blew, where the brick chimneys belched the roiling plumes of progress, and where the long-bearded Jews in skullcaps, round glasses, and long black gabardines tussled over theological questions like crows fighting over pieces of bread.

Like most of the Jews, particularly the Jews who didn't own the factories, Frances and her family lived in the slums of Baluty, thousands of them packed in the basements or in garrets of dilapidated houses like herring in dockside crates. In all of Poland, only Warsaw had a larger Jewish population than Lødz; nearly half the city's 410,000 people in 1910 were Jews. Flat-faced, stone tenements, two or three stories high, hugged the narrow streets that wound through the city in a maze of dark, narrow hallways—streets now sprinkled with Russian soldiers.

It wasn't supposed to be like this. Regina's husband, Dawid, had left for America two springs before, knowing full well that she was going to have the baby, but also knowing full well that Poland, for the Jews, would forever be more prison than home. He and Regina had both been born in 1881, the year the *pogroms* slaughtered Jews in villages across the pale. On ponies, the Cossacks swooped into villages at night like dogs ripped free from their leashes. They swept across Poland, torching synagogues. They shattered Stars of David symbols with their swords—*Hep, hep Jude!* They killed and maimed and laughed as they rode off into the darkness, their vodka-fueled violence triggered by well-worn stories of Jews murdering Christian children.

New edicts were issued that robbed the Jews of the right to live in a particular place, to gain an education, to earn a living. Exiled, the Jews trudged toward cities such as Lødz to begin anew, everything they owned piled in carts or strapped to their backs. But the hatred followed them. Shortly after Dawid and Regina married in Lødz, the Revolution of 1905 sparked a new wave of vengeance against the Jews. It reached a crescendo in

1912 when the Jews voted for the "wrong candidate" in an election. They paid the price in blood.

Enough. Others had left for America. Why not the Schlangers? Dawid had a cousin, Jacob Grossman, in a place called Boston, Massachusetts. He had offered Dawid room in his flat on Harrison Avenue. Dawid figured that within a year he could earn enough money to bring his wife and children to America. He arrived at Ellis Island on May 22, 1913, aboard the steamship *Pretoria*, having turned thirty-two years old just two days out of New York Harbor. Once in Boston, he began work as a fruit peddler.

Three months later, back in Lødz, Regina gave birth to Freidel Yachet Schlanger. To the Poles, she was a Jew and, thus, a threat. To the Jews, she was a girl and, thus, a liability. "Many daughters, many troubles," went the Jewish saying. "Many sons, many honors." To Dawid she was a name that arrived in a letter and, thus, an unknown. But to her mother, Freidel was a *shayna maidel*—a beautiful girl, her blessed second daughter. Freidel was a brown-eyed, brown-haired babe whom Regina honored with the Yiddish name *Faiga* after the baby's paternal grandmother, Frajda Górska.

The following June, in 1914, Dawid was close to having earned enough money for his family's passage to America when the news hit Lødz's Piotrkow Street: in Sarajevo, the capital of Bosnia, Archduke Franz Ferdinand, heir to the throne of Austria-Hungary, had been assassinated by a Bosnian Serb. Like a lightning strike on a tinder-dry forest, World War I exploded. And Regina's worst fears soon came to pass: with German submarines prowling the Atlantic Ocean's shipping lanes, steamship owners decided the passage to America was too dangerous to risk under any flag. Immigration ground to a halt.

Thus did Freidel Schlanger begin her life: no more free than the hardened streams that only weeks before had flowed into Poland's Vistula River but were now frozen in place by forces beyond themselves.

As NOVEMBER deepened, the icy breath of war chilled the neck of Lødz. German troops—250,000 of them—advanced north by train as winter hardened the lifeless plains in a sea of white. In and around Lødz, some 150,000 Russian troops braced for the attack. In the Schlanger family's drafty flat, amid coughs and sniffles, Regina huddled Chaja and Freidel close, her body far warmer than their straw beds. Around them: relatives, bound by blood and, for now, a common fear that deepened with the sound in the distance. Cannons began pounding. It was November 18, 1914. The Battle of Lødz had begun.

The two forces clashed on the city's fringes, and occasionally in the city itself, day after bitter day. Temperatures dipped to 10 degrees Fahrenheit. Soldiers froze to death in trenches while trying to sleep. "The battlefield was swimming in blood," reported *The Times* of London. "Discarded German capes, Prayer-books, notebooks, gaiters, gloves, cartridge boxes, haversacks, gnawed bones, tinned meat cans, and straw from the trenches littered the hill slopes. Deep pits had been made by shells in front of the trenches, and in the trenches were heaps of corpses. From the battlefield, Lødz appeared to be enveloped in red flames, and several fires occurred daily in the town. Parts of the cities had been shelled. The people were defenceless."

After nearly three weeks of fighting, the Russians fell back and reorganized their line. But Germany's victory was costly. When the battle was over, Germany had suffered 35,000 casualties, the Russians considerably more. But the other losers wore no uniforms at all. They were people like Regina Schlanger and her daughters who now lived in a city that belonged to someone else: Germany. Few citizens had been killed or wounded in actual battle. Many were, or would one day become, casualties of a different kind.

The capture of Lødz would be only a prelude to far greater German dominance in the future. In fact, the newborn sons of these German soldiers—sons born in Germany this same year and essentially the same age as Freidel Schlanger—would some-day be stamped with a mark of national German nobility. Twenty-one years hence, they would become Adolf Hitler's first conscripted military class. During World War II, some would wind up fighting in the hedgerows of Normandy or on the Eastern Front. Others would wind up working in a quaint tourist village 120 miles south of Lødz, a 700-year-old town where tourists visited to see castles, churches, and synagogues, and stopped to enjoy a cup of tea at the Hotel Herz. Its name was Oswiecim. But in time it would be better known by its German moniker: Auschwitz.

AFTER THE BATTLE, the once-vibrant city lay still, like a frozen animal left in the wake of a snowstorm. People walked around in a daze, some having lost fortunes, others jobs, others family members to the typhoid fever that had broken out. Regina broke off pieces of dry bread and gave them to Chaja and Freidel; later, thanks to a local relief agency, she would get a quart of cabbage soup to feed the three of them for a day.

Water pumps froze. To get water, Regina would melt snow on a meager fire, fueled by whatever wood scraps she could find in a city so desperate that people had ripped down the fence around the New Jewish Cemetery and burned it in their apart-ments. At night, when the cold awakened her, Regina broke the ice that would form in the jug of water so her daughters would have something to drink come morning.

The Schlangers' experience was virtually everyone's experience in Lødz. Regina and her daughters waited in food-ration lines while the horse-drawn carts rolled down the street carrying the German wounded, their uniforms dirty, their bodies splotched with the dry, crusted blood of war, their eyes looking into nothingness. This was the childhood Freidel Schlanger knew. "The poor, half-mad women run after you, seize you by the sleeves, and gaze at you with inflamed eyes," wrote a *Times* correspondent, "while the children follow them, swollen faces livid from the cold."

In weeks to come, German soldiers, wearing formed-leather helmets with brass spikes on top and wrapped in woolen greatcoats, swaggered from flat to flat. Freidel heard the soldiers bang on the door with the butts of their rifles and watched them kick it open with their knee-high jackboots. Freidel and her aunts and uncles and cousins cowered together. The soldiers entered and took what they pleased: copper pots and brass door-knobs and menorahs. Whatever might be melted down and used for ammunition. Whatever war demanded.

Tuberculosis and typhoid fever epidemics broke out. Hospitals were too crowded to handle all the afflicted people. Hordes of paupers were hauled off to disinfecting stations to be scrubbed, shaved, and deloused. Soldiers mocked the Jewish poor as they were stripped for scrubbings. As weeks became months, Regina hung on to her monthly ration card as if it were made of gold. But her paltry diet diluted whatever nutrients she might pass on to Freidel through her milk. She'd all but forgotten the taste of potato cakes or hot chickpeas. For two weeks, Lødz had no bread at all. For months, no meat.

Meanwhile, the streets became the property of funeral processions. Unemployed women sold their bodies for a crust of bread. Some others offered their children to employers in exchange for something to eat or forced the boys and girls to become food smugglers. In Baluty, the weak sounds of Sabbath songs endured, an occasional violin softening the hard edges of hopelessness. The gossips lost their zeal for Baluty's smut. Instead, they whispered of unspeakable horrors that they'd heard from faraway families, like the bayoneted bodies of children outside Lødz. *Have you heard? They were hung on fences like scarecrows!*

Finally, the spring of 1915 arrived, bringing with it not the usual smell of plowed fields and fresh vegetables, but the whiff of thawed sewers—and the rancid stench of thawed bodies from the battlefields beyond. For four years, Germany and Russia took turns sucking life out of a once-vibrant city and its once-vibrant people, whether that meant plundering houses, retooling factories for the war effort, hoarding food for themselves, or ripping the beards off Orthodox Jews.

At war's end, in 1918, foreign delegations arrived in the region to assess the damage. They disagreed as to whether Germans or Russians were responsible for the horror left behind, but this they agreed on: nowhere in eastern Europe was the suffering of civilians during World War I greater than in Lødz, Poland. Wrote one American journalist: "All that [is] left are the graves of the dead, the emaciated bodies of the living, and the shell-scarred land, denuded of almost every trace of vegetation."

Freidel Schlanger was nearly five years old when World War I ended. She was gaunt, with dark, hollow eyes that had seen far too much. But alive.

AT 7:30 A.M., the *Pendleton's* engines stopped. By now, the drone had become so rote in the ears of the hundreds onboard that the new silence held an eerie foreboding, especially when punctuated by the sound of German shells lobbed into the flotilla from gun emplacements beyond the beach.

Frances awoke. She pulled out a French phrase book she'd been issued in England. Not all of the wounded they'd be treating would be soldiers; some would be French civilians. A few bunks away, the heart of a fellow nurse, Betty Belanger, pounded harder. Every shell or stray machine-gun bullet from a German plane seemed to ping closer and closer to the twenty-five-year-old nurse from Manchester, New Hampshire.

Above many of the ships in the Allied armada, silvery, fat, barrage balloons floated ghostlike in the sky, tethered to the ships to dissuade low-flying aerial attacks by the *Luftwaffe*. The balloons hadn't done much dissuading this particular morning. One merchant marine ship, the *Charles Morgan*, had been sunk by a *Luftwaffe* bomb and at 4:15 A.M., a glider bomb exploded in the water beside the *Pendleton*. The shell's impact buckled a bulkhead, caused an oil leak into a water tank, and reminded those on board that they weren't back in bucolic England anymore.

In Upton-on-Severn, the English town where the Forty-fifth had been billeted for most of its time before leaving for France, the nurses had spent time at hand-driven sewing machines, making giant "Geneva" red crosses out of bed sheets. One nurse would turn the sewing-machine's wheel while another fed a sheet through.

"What is this for?" Sallylou had asked when first hearing of the task.

"We'll put the crosses on the tents and in the field next to us," explained Capt. Elizabeth Hay, the Forty-fifth's chief nurse, "so the German airplanes won't target us."

Sallylou frowned ever so slightly. Until then, she hadn't given serious thought to the idea that their lives might be in danger. But if the lessons of war seemed far away in England, they were now getting closer. On the ship, soldiers repositioned themselves on their bunks again and again. "How long till we go?" The question passed from stem to stern and back like a subway rumor. The consensus: *A helluva lot longer than we think . . .*

An hour . . . Maybe ten . . . Maybe never . . . After all, weren't we supposed to have gone in yesterday, at Omaha?

The *Pendleton*, whose passenger list also included nurses from the 128th Evacuation Hospital, had left Falmouth, near England's farthest southwest reaches, at 2:30 A.M. Thursday, June 8. But after the 100-mile journey, the vessel was wrongly positioned off Omaha Beach and the error had cost the ship a full day in repositioning.

Meanwhile, soldiers had been kept in the dark about what was happening in France. They knew the basics: Hitler's troops had spent four years fortifying the French coast with their vaunted "Atlantic Wall" to defend territory Germany had occupied since 1940. The wall had fallen on D-Day. But to win back Europe, Allied troops now had to defeat the Germans. And that meant bringing ashore more than ten times as many men as had landed on June 6, which is why the soldiers below now awaited the command to board landing craft, hit the beaches, and join the cause of liberation. At stake? As simple as it was agonizingly complex: the freedom of the world.

Though some had heard erroneous BBC radio reports suggesting the D-Day invasion had been made with "surprising ease," most knew better. "What worries me about landing," said one commander of a ship heading across the English Channel, "is the bomb holes the Air Force may leave in the beach before we hit. The chart may show three feet of water, but the men may step into a ten-foot hole anywhere."

Once ashore, the nurses were to rendezvous with the men of the Forty-fifth's 226-person unit, who were arriving on a different transport to preclude an entire outfit from being lost should the Germans sink the ship. From Utah Beach, the Forty-fifth would divide into three platoons and, with help from veteran doctors who'd finished surgical stints in North Africa, leapfrog across France, patching the wounded.

As the *Pendleton* bobbed on anchor, stomachs grew queasy, palms moist—these weren't sailors used to the chop of the sea, or, for that matter, the idea of fighting a war. Lying on her bunk, Frances fidgeted in her wool uniform; a gunnysack, she figured, would be less scratchy. The whole getup had been designed, and sized, for men, not women: a wool uniform that hung on the nurses like tree moss, a field jacket, and "coveralls" coated with some ungodly waxy substance—it looked like axle grease—that was supposed to protect against mustard gas. For now, the grease simply made Frances stink, itch, and sweat. Canvas leggings connected the uniform to man-sized boots, akin to wearing a couple of leather anchors. Finally, when called to go, Frances and the others would wrap life belts around their waists, complete with a couple of rubber tubes used to inflate the flotation devices. The ensemble made Frances and her fellow nurses resemble snow-day kids bundled up by overprotective moms.

She twisted her short-cropped hair into spit curls, securing them with bobby pins. A hairnet would go over her head, then the helmet: Each nurse had been issued a steel helmet, supposedly strong enough to deflect most shrapnel but not a direct hit from a bullet. Each helmet had a single gold bar painted on the front to signify the wearer's status as a second lieutenant. Each nurse wore a red cross on a white band, wrapped and pinned to her left arm. The latter, supposedly, would signal to the Germans that this person—as per the Geneva Convention—was not to be targeted. Alas, those in the Forty-fifth would soon learn that the rules of war were sometimes broken.

The ship's bell rang every half hour. Eleven bells came, then twelve noon, then 1 P.M. The bunks in the ship's hold—more like glorified stretchers—rolled with the sea. Nerves tightened, wound by the tedious passing of time and the wondering of the unknown. Beads of condensation formed on the steel ceilings, then dripped on soldiers and nurses below.

Suddenly, with petrifying urgency, the bosun's whistle sounded and the ship's loudspeaker squawked to life. "Now hear this! Now hear this! All troops to your debarkation areas! All troops to your debarkation areas!" Frances stuffed her notebook in a musette bag and donned her oversized helmet.

The time had come. It was shortly before 2 P.M. on June 10, 1944. Everywhere, soldiers and nurses ran through last-minute mental checklists. Frances zipped, then buttoned her field jacket and fastened her canvas life belt. Soldiers double-checked their M-1 Garand rifles, carbines, and Thompson submachine guns. Then, guts churning from a sickening blend of nausea and fear, they all filed through the ship's narrow passageways, up to the windswept deck, and toward whatever lay beyond.

CHAPTER 2

*There was a dream . . . that men could one day speak the
thoughts of their own choosing. There was a hope . . . that
men could one day stroll through the streets unafraid. There
was a prayer . . . that each could speak to his own God—in
his own church. That dream, that hope, that prayer
became . . . America.*

—ANONYMOUS,
FOUND IN FRANCES SLANGER'S CHAPBOOK

Aboard the *Pendleton*, Frances Slanger and the Forty-fifth
Field Hospital's nurses huddled on the vomit-slicked main
deck, a place both freeing and frightening. The nurses had been
belowdecks so long that they felt liberated by the fresh air. Every
direction they looked, the English Channel was dotted with
ships ferrying Allied troops to France. Momentarily, Frances was
lost in the magnitude of the moment, all of it bathed in bright
sunshine. Suddenly, a German 88-millimeter cannon shell
parted the air with the sound of ripped canvas. Bombs exploded
near the ship, sending occasional shrapnel on deck. Frances
looked around: Soldiers flitted this way and that. Some gathered
around a chaplain who offered hasty prayers and blessings. Some
slickened the deck with their upchucked breakfasts.

"Over here, Forty-fifth!" yelled Capt. Elizabeth Hay, a large woman in her mid-forties, far older than the rest but only slightly less scared. Only a day before, Hay's fears were that her nurses would try to sneak canteen coffee from the mess hall (which they did, and were promptly caught) or, worse, that enlisted men would infiltrate beyond the black curtains that had been hung between her nurses and the 90 percent of the ship that was male (which they didn't). Now, the trivial seemed even more so.

The nurses stood more than three stories above a landing craft that was reachable only by a cargo net hung over the ship's side. The rock of the ship and a stiff wind whipped the net. Frances looked over the port rail to the waiting landing craft. It was, she realized, considerably farther down than Oneida Street was from the rooftop writing perch she'd carved out back home in Boston. She gave a quick study to the faces of the women to her right and left: Belanger, Montague, Cummings, Bowler, "Tex," and a dozen others. They showed no less worry than hers, a fact that was equal parts assuring (she wasn't the only one about to wet her fatigues) and unsettling (how were they going to make it into that boat below?).

What was that sailor's quote she'd pasted in her chapbook? "Small skill is gained by those who cling to ease;/The able sailor hails from stormy seas." But had its author ever been under aerial attack while trying to climb down a 40-foot rope ladder? Still, as another shell exploded near the ship, leaving the *Pendleton* looked like the lesser of two evils from Frances's perspective. With shells pounding, the Forty-fifth might as well be standing in the middle of a bull's-eye. A landing craft was at least a smaller target, and a moving one as well.

"Let's go!" yelled Hay above the roar of wind, planes, and artillery. "Go, girls, go, go, go!" Burdened by garb and gear, musette bags slung over one shoulder and gas masks clipped to neck harnesses, Frances Slanger and the other nurses started down the thirty-foot netting. They'd survived obstacle courses at training back in the States, but nothing like this one. The ship rose and fell. One slip and a nurse was, at best, badly injured. At worst, dead on arrival.

Frances and the other seventeen nurses headed down the rope ladder, faces to the ships, backs to the sea. Once even with the LCVP (Landing Craft, Vehicle and Personnel), the women were to time their jumps to coincide with the top of a swell to shorten the distance of the fall. On D-Day, four days earlier, many soldiers had failed; more than two dozen had suffered broken legs in the first hour of debarkation alone and at least three were crushed to death when caught between ships and landing craft.

Sallylou Cummings made it. Betty Belanger made it. Mae Montague, a nurse from Woonsocket, Rhode Island, made it. Frances inched her way to the net's bottom, then, eyes frozen in fear, turned to look at the waiting boat, rising and falling with the pitch of the sea.

"Come on, Frances," Cummings yelled. "You can do it. Jump!"

The ship and landing craft rose and fell, Frances's confidence along with them. She clung tight to two horizontal sections of ropes, her boots balancing wobbly on two others beneath her. *Remember the training exercises, remember the training exercises . . .*

"Let's go, Slanger!" yelled Captain Hay.

Frances mustered whatever grit she had inside, then leapt, falling into the arms of the fellow nurses amid a burst of cheers. All eighteen nurses soon were aboard.

The Coast Guard coxswain at the helm steered the landing craft on its ten-mile journey to Utah Beach. Crammed together, Frances and the other nurses stood shoulder to shoulder like shotgun shells in a box. They couldn't see out; the gunwales were too high. They listened to the deep-throated thrum of the engines and the occasional boom of distant artillery. The square-faced ramp of the assault craft butted forward through the swells.

Utah Beach, like the four other landing beaches code-named by the Allies, had been secured by American troops early on D-Day. In part because those troops mistakenly landed down the beach from what turned out to be a heavily defended stretch of coastline, Utah hadn't been the bloodbath that Omaha Beach had been twelve miles southeast. At Omaha, waves lapped over dead GIs in shallows turned a muddy pink by their blood. And yet soldiers, more than 200, had died at Utah Beach, too. Ships had been blown apart by mines. More than a dozen landing craft had gone down.

"Remember, straight lines!" yelled Captain Hay. "And watch for shell holes!"

The nurses glanced around at one another. Most were twenty-five to thirty years old. All were registered nurses. All but Hay were single. While in England, the staging area for the invasion of France, Sallylou Cummings had met a handsome young doctor from North Dakota named John Bonzer. Now, she wondered where the young man with the apple-rose cheeks was in this sprawling flotilla. Mae "Monty" Montague, a blue-eyed, brown-haired nurse, felt her dog-tag chain to make sure her new engagement ring was still there; she'd gotten engaged at Camp Kilmer on the last night before the Forty-fifth had shipped out. Her fiancé, Ed Bowen, was an administrative officer with the unit's Third Platoon. As his promise, he'd given her his Salisbury State (Maryland) College ring until he could find something better.

Beside Monty stood Dottie Richter of Dover, Delaware. Six months before, she had sauntered into North Carolina's Fort Bragg fresh from a powder-puff, regular army assignment in Puerto Rico, golf clubs on one shoulder, tennis racket in her hand. "*My,*" Monty had said at the time, "what have we *here?*" Now, aboard the landing craft, Dottie swallowed hard.

Next to Dottie, Elizabeth Powers, of Lowell, Massachusetts, cupped a hand over her nose and mouth so she wouldn't inhale any more direct diesel fumes. With the other, she searched her field jacket for that standard army issue: "Bag, vomit, one."

Amid the stench of diesel, Frances discerned the faint puffs of brine coming off the ocean. She took a deep breath. She closed her eyes. Her life had been, was now, and would forever be marked by the comings and goings of ships at sea.

ABOARD THE IMMIGRANT SHIP, *Nieuw Amsterdam*, deep in the fetid darkness of the steerage compartment, mothers suckled crying babies. Passengers played cards, prayed, slept, and smoked. Mostly, though, they waited, and wondered aloud in Yiddish: Could they bear another five days of this?

Regina Schlanger put her hand to Freidel's chin and gently tilted her daughter's head back. She was doing it again: looking at the swollen eye. Now seven, Freidel had developed an eye infection shortly before they'd boarded the windowless train in Łødz headed to Rotterdam, Holland, for the crossing to America. Because steamship companies bore the return-trip expenses of immigrants turned back at Ellis Island, it was in their best interest to conduct thorough examinations of their potential passengers. Still, European exams tended to be brief, for which Regina Schlanger thanked God. Freidel had been given a cursory look and allowed to board.

By now, the Ellis Island stories had made their way through steerage like a fever. Stories about how some passengers were rejected and sent back to their homelands. About the new literacy tests, designed specifically to cut down on the number of immigrants that were allowed in. About how World War I had chilled the hearts of Americans toward foreigners, who worried that Eastern Europeans were all Bolsheviks—and, thus, suspect.

Vellin zay luzzin oonts ahrine? The Yiddish phrase weaved through the masses in steerage each day. *Will America let us in?*

On their eleventh day at sea, passengers aboard the 615-foot *Nieuw Amsterdam* were allowed on deck. There they saw a thin strip of land in the distance. Fear gave way to excitement; they were getting closer to the *goldene medineh*, the golden land. And the next morning, when the ship sliced through The Narrows, hearts pounded. There, rising from the waters, was the "Great Lady" of which they had heard: the Statue of Liberty. Taking the hands of Chaja and Freidel, Regina scrambled to the port rail, trying vainly to get a peek for herself and for her daughters. Passengers cheered. Hats flew in the air. People hugged and wept—all because of the sight of the woman whose torch was proudly thrust upward, offering light for those who'd known so little of it.

Regina, head wrapped in a scarf, basked in the moment with gratitude, though she couldn't completely lose herself in celebration. It was Freidel's eye. Though she wanted to believe otherwise, Regina couldn't help but notice something during the twelve-day journey: The eye had gotten worse.

A LIGHT RAINSTORM swept up the northeast seaboard on the morning of September 7, 1920, bringing showers to New York Harbor and beyond. But the rain wasn't enough to scrub the Yankees–Philadelphia Athletics baseball game at the Polo Grounds, nor enough to muffle the excitement of immigrants readying to leave the *Nieuw Amsterdam* as the ship anchored off Ellis Island.

Once the ship was moored, immigration officials boarded to give first- and second-class passengers a cursory inspection. A more arduous process awaited those in steerage, who comprised 2,200 of the *Nieuw Amsterdam*'s 2,846 passengers. Some were

Czechoslovakians and Germans. Most, however, were Polish Jews, passengers with names such as Grendla Katz, Netti Schaffer, Sara Sirota, Breina Levi, Josef Wrabel, and Anna Mistnik. Women outnumbered men two to one, many husbands, such as Dawid, having already gone to America to secure work or having been killed in the war. And they were often large families: the *Nieuw Amsterdam* was full of families with half a dozen people or more.

Along with other steerage passengers, Regina and her girls were loaded on a barge and taken to Ellis Island. One by one the immigrants stepped onto American soil for the first time: women wrapped in scarves and shawls and wearing whatever "best" outfit they had, thinking it might make the difference between their family being allowed to enter; bearded and mustachioed men in felt hats and wool suits shouldering bags and dragging travel-worn trunks; and hundreds of children, like Freidel and Chaja.

On the gangway, Freidel walked across this bridge to America, the tall buildings stretching skyward beyond. Around her she saw trunks, straw baskets, and suitcases stuffed so tightly that they looked like mothers ready to give birth. She saw people wearing multiple sweaters and jackets because each item was one less item they had to carry. Some of the larger women, dark skirts hanging to the ground, shuffled along with the look of human bells.

Freidel held tightly to her mother's hand. Around her swirled hundreds of conversations in numerous languages, blending together in a cacophony of chatter, like blackbirds thick in a tree. The immigrants may have been haggard and sick from twelve days of eating haddock, their skin tinted ever-so-slightly green from the pitch and roll of the ship. They may have been sore, smelly, and mentally dulled. But they tingled with emotion. Though burdened with fear, they were also alive with expectations.

Freidel knew the feeling. She was, after all, perhaps soon to meet the *tateh*—the father—she had never met. What would he look like? *Be* like? What would he think of her? What would she think of him?

The mass of people inched forward, into a giant building where their baggage was checked, then headed up a flight of stairs to what was known as "The Great Registry Room." Freidel clung to Regina, just as she had done back home when the soldiers had come. Save for the prayers she'd been taught, her mother was her only security.

Freidel looked around at a room larger than any she had ever seen. It had an arched ceiling, red tile floor, and rows of wooden benches. Two American flags hung prominently high above both ends of the rectangular-shaped hall—huge, bright patterns of red, white, and blue. Below: dirty, sweaty, tired immigrants, some asleep on their baggage, others hot with fever. The smell of backed-up toilets drifted across the room. The line toward the physical inspections snaked back and forth, people being pushed and prodded by immigrant officials, some of whom would gladly allow a young, pretty woman passage—for favors later, that is.

Ellis Island had woefully underestimated the glut of post–World War I immigrants. Ventilation was poor and only six bathtubs were available for women and small children. "Why should I fear the fires of hell?" an immigrant had etched on an Ellis Island wall. "I have been through Ellis Island."

It had become known as the "Island of Hope" and the "Island of Tears." And Freidel would soon understood why.

By now it was early afternoon and Freidel hadn't eaten since early morning. She felt someone touch her. She turned to find a strange woman pinning a felt number on her wool jacket, her "manifest" number. Everyone got a number like this. Little was said to her or to her mother by immigration officials, who had no idea which of a dozen-plus languages the newcomers might speak. Gestures were made, fingers pointed, heads nodded. Signs were all but meaningless. The language barrier was steep.

Regina fanned herself and the girls as the waiting continued. The high in New York on this late-summer day would be only 77 degrees, but inside the Ellis Island building, temperatures climbed far beyond. As people were called into the medical examination rooms, those who waited slid down the benches, repeating the procedure time and again as the day dragged on.

Amid the confusion, even a seven-year-old like Freidel would realize what was happening: some people were being allowed to pass and some were not. Immigrants couldn't miss seeing "the mark." The first doctor would look at the newcomers in general. The immigrants were asked to say something, then to drop their trousers or lift their dresses, sometimes in view of other passengers. If there was anything at all suspicious about a patient, a doctor would reach for the chalk. An "H" would indicate heart trouble. An "X" would flag a mental disorder. An "E"—eye trouble. When a case aroused suspicion, the immigrant was temporarily placed in a cage, away from the rest.

Regina and her daughters inched forward. Freidel grew afraid when a female doctor—women and girls were usually examined by women—took her mother aside for an examination. For a girl who had clung to her mother for thousands of miles, a few feet of separation was traumatic, even though the doctors did it this way to ease the fear of the child's own exam.

When the doctor had finished with her mother and with Chaja, she turned to Freidel. Immediately, she began examining Freidel's swollen eye with that same squinty-eye look that her mother had used, tilting the girl's head this way and that, as if something were wrong. She reached for a light and shined it in one of Freidel's eyes, then the other. She reached for a tongue depressor to check in Freidel's mouth. And then, Freidel's eyes widened like a horse who's seen a snake: the woman in the white dress reached for the chalk. She scrawled something on Freidel's shoulder. It was the letter "E."

Above a room already humming with conversation, you can imagine a mother's Yiddish cry: *Nein, nein, nicht mein tochter! Nicht mein tochter!* But it was Regina's daughter, and she was being taken away from her. Freidel grabbed her mother's hand. Regina grabbed her daughter's. The nurse gently but firmly separated the two, having done this hundreds of times before. Freidel looked back, not wanting to face whatever lay ahead, her eyes wet with tears. She was placed in the wire cage with others who were being detained.

Mama! Mama!

Until now, Freidel had never been apart from her mother. She broke into tears. Despite being in a room packed with dozens of others, she was alone, separated from the only stability she'd known. A doctor or nurse may well have done her best to assure Freidel not to worry, but the words were not words the little girl understood—and the affirming touches on her shoulders were not from familiar hands. She wanted to be back with Mama and Chaja.

Freidel wilted. She was, in this moment, powerless: a seven-year-old Jewish girl whose life was in the hands of others. A child with no voice, no standing, no country, and, for the moment, no family. Outside, in New York Harbor, ships boldly headed out to sea, billowed with pride and purpose. Inside, huddled in a ball, face stained with tears, Freidel Schlanger cowered like a wounded bird.

A BOARD OF INQUIRY had the ultimate decision about who passed through Ellis Island, but if doctors chose to exclude an immigrant because of disease the board was bound to accept that choice. In other words, if a single doctor believed Freidel's eye infection was disease-related and sufficiently serious to turn her away, her fate was sealed. There would be no second opinion, no hearing, no appeal. No chance for Regina to speak with an official through an interpreter. No chance to plead her daughter's case, to explain how Freidel was a good girl, how she made her mother proud, and how if this new country—this so-called land of opportunity—would grant the little girl passage, she would make America proud.

Finally, they came for Freidel—a small group of doctors. They reexamined her. They huddled, saying words that she could not understand—and could barely hear over the din of hundreds of conversations elsewhere. Their heads nodded up and down, then sideways. What did this mean? Regina waited down the hall, praying for *gutteh nahyees*—good news—from the doctors.

Across the harbor, David Slanger—he'd had his name changed from Dawid Schlanger since coming to America—looked toward Ellis Island amid a throng of others. This ship, Regina had said in the letter, was the one she and the girls would be on. But where were they—the wife he had not seen in seven years, the daughter whom he'd left as a little girl and would now be a young woman, and this new one, the one called Freidel?

Freidel, shaking, was taken from the cage and down a hallway. *Mama!* Freidel wrapped her arms around the bent-over woman. An interpreter said something to Regina. That's when Freidel saw the same look on her mother's face that she'd seen when Mama had rushed her and Chaja to the ship's deck to see the tall woman with the torch: a huge smile, not something she saw often on her mother's face. Now, in the medical area, her mother hugged her close, then gathered Chaja into the fold.

Dee ducktoyrem zug'n oz zay vel'n dir a'reinluzn tsu Amerikeh! They would allow Freidel entry into America.

After the three were ferried across the Harbor, Freidel saw

her new *tateh*, or father, who was waiting for them. He was not as tall as she had imagined he would be. His coat smelled of cigarette smoke. She could tell because he had bent down to hug her, this man whom she had never seen before. It seemed odd, hugging a stranger; until now, she had hugged only her mother and, when saying good-bye at the train station in Lødz, her aunts, uncles, and cousins. And yet it also seemed good.

The four of them, linked by arms and hands, walked toward the train station, away from the "Great Lady," New York Harbor, and the waters that no longer separated them.

IN THE LIGHT SWELLS off Normandy, the gray landing craft neared the beach. Frances checked the adjustable band in her helmet; it never seemed tight enough and her helmet was forever tilting to the side. The moment was coming. Once they hit the beach, the eighteen nurses would join the men and split into three seventy-five-person platoons. Frances was part of the Second Platoon. Then they'd begin following the troops east toward Germany, tending to the wounded in field hospital tents.

As Frances braced for the landing, she was about to fulfill what Col. Oveta Culp Hobby, the director of the Women's Army Corps, had once told a batch of recruits: "You have taken off silk and put on khaki. You have a debt and a date. A debt to democracy and a date with destiny."

Frances Slanger believed being part of the Army Nurse Corps was the most important job she'd ever done. America, at large, however, was far more skeptical about her being in the military than she was. Only as war in Europe loomed did some commanders warm to the idea of having women part of the U.S. military. In general, soldiers' reactions ranged from enthusiasm to amusement to flat-out hostility. Newspapers and magazines, even ones published by the military such as *Yank*, looked at army nurses with a sort of "wink-wink" brush-off.

"Warmly, yet stylishly dressed are these army nurses who stop to frolic on the way to a luncheon . . ." read the caption beneath a *Boston Globe* photo in 1944. *Yank* magazine would run a feature on gallant soldiers in Italy next to a story on summer wear for women in the military. In the media's eye, nurses in uniform were curiosities who made good copy—mascots who traveled with the team and added a certain spice to things, but weren't really part of the game itself.

Reporters, even many female reporters, focused far more on *who* the nurses were—"girls"—than *what* they did. Cartoonists had a field day with bras and bosoms and "petticoat army" quips. The public at large was even less kind. Rumors abounded that women in the armed services were either uniformed hussies out to steal husbands and boyfriends, or were lesbians.

As U.S. involvement in World War II deepened, the military realized that it had been naive in thinking that all able-bodied military men wanted to see action. Some, in fact, preferred the safety of Stateside. But women—350,000 would serve in World War II—often freed those Stateside soldiers to fight, which drew resentment toward those women from soldiers and their families.

On the cusp of battle in the European Theater of Operations, some soldiers looked at the nurses with a touch of resentment but most men were more curious than disdainful. Some of the military's 60,000 army nurses were beautiful; some were not. But they did a job that men didn't do—male nurses, in fact, weren't allowed in the Army Nurse Corps—and so weren't threatening to most soldiers. Besides, they were American women whose job it was to help sick and wounded men get better, and in the eyes of a soldier, that alone counted for something.

The landing craft ground to a halt on the sandy bottom,

about 600 feet from shore. The waiting was over. Frances and the seventeen other nurses of the Forty-fifth pushed toward the bow ramp. The gate ratcheted down with an ominous rattle of chains. And, as she'd done twenty-three years before, Frances Slanger saw before her a new country that would change her life forever.

"Let's go!" yelled Captain Hay. "Go, go, go! Com'n, girls!" One by one, the nurses of the Forty-fifth splashed down, musette bags held over their heads, life belts on, but, in these shallow waters, not inflated. Along with those of the 128th Evacuation Hospital, they were the first U.S. nurses to hit the Normandy beach after D-Day.

The surf was light. Frances took one final look at shore—a fuzzy look since she'd pocketed her glasses—then at the waters below. It was only three to four feet deep but, in terms of height, she wasn't exactly "Tiny" Schwartz, her six-foot-three friend. Frances paused for a moment, held tight to her musette bag, then jumped. The cold jolted her. It was like the Cape Cod water she'd experienced—but in *December*. Because of her shortness, the water came up higher on her than it did on the others—to her chest, and higher when waves rolled past her. As if in slow motion, Frances tried to build forward momentum amid water that, one moment, worked for her, the next moment against. The blurred beach was 200 yards away. Most nurses began reaching the shallows and, ultimately, the beach. But, up ahead, Betty Belanger, four inches taller than Frances, was having a hard time finding her balance. Seeing the corpse of a GI being toyed by the surf did nothing for her confidence. She had to be helped ashore.

Likewise, near the end of the pack, Frances wobbled unsteadily. She struggled to find forward momentum, but, in an eyeblink, was suddenly gone. Beneath the water's surface, she thrashed her arms and legs, the smooth, sandy bottom having given way to the deep pock of a shell hole. The weight of her boots, three-pound life belt, and three-pound helmet worked against her. A few nurses suddenly realized she'd disappeared. So did some of the waiting GIs who'd been helping nurses ashore.

"Frances!" yelled Sallylou. Her voice ratcheted to panic level. "Frances!"

Frances Slanger twisted in a vortex of bubbles and fear, fighting to get her head back above water. The salt water stung her eyes. Briefly, she came up for a desperate gulp of air. But as quickly as she had surfaced, she once again disappeared into the Normandy waters and their hunger for the dead. She wanted to keep fighting—*had* to keep fighting—but after a few seconds of underwater struggle, such resolve tilted toward resignation. That's when she felt them: hands dragging her upward. Blessed, out-of-nowhere hands. As it turned out, GI hands.

Frances Slanger grabbed two soldiers' arms and hung on. Her head broke the surface. She spewed out the salt water and gasped. Her boots once again touched sand.

"Y' OK, Slanger?" asked Sallylou.

In chest-high water, Frances gulped, nodded a frantic "yes," found her footing on the bottom, and lurched forward. She was cold. She was disoriented. But she was alive.

"Head for the bank!" yelled one of the Forty-fifth's officers, Capt. William Poe, who was standing up to his knees in the shallows. "Let's go, girls—fast!"

Poe, an administrative officer from St. Louis with deep-chiseled features, had come in a day earlier to organize the Forty-fifth when it arrived. He was tired, unshaven, and cranky. "Krauts gave us hell last night," he said to Cummings. Down the beach, just offshore, the landing craft that the Forty-fifth's men were on was delaying its arrival because of heavy fire from inland emplacements.

A shell whistled overhead and exploded down the beach

from the nurses, sending sand, water, and shrapnel into the air. A German plane strafed the beach with machine-gun fire. The sound of surf was lost in the roar of weapons, vehicles, and soldiers. Sallylou took one look and thought: *What in God's name are we doing here?* So much for starched nurses' caps, white uniforms, and navy blue capes. Frances half-ran and half-walked up the beach, dragging behind her the water-weighted musette bag that some GI had retrieved from the surf. The smell of diesel blended with the stench of her gas-impregnated coveralls and smoke that hung over the beach.

"Hey, will ya get a load of that!" yelled some GI. The word spread quickly, triggering cheers, hand claps, and scattered cat calls. "Nurses! Hey guys, we got nurses!"

AT NEARLY the same hour that the Forty-fifth's nurses had debarked from the *Pendleton* into the landing craft, a young Frenchman strode purposefully down the main street cobblestones of Oradour-sur-Glane, about 250 miles southeast of Normandy. He had a bouquet of daisies in his hand.

"*Bonjour,*" said Albert Roumbi to a passerby, a bit more lilt in his voice than usual.

The time had come. It was shortly before 2 P.M. on June 10, 1944. On this day, he would look deeply into the eyes of his true love and say the words he'd been mulling for some time: *Veux-tu m'épouser?* On this day he was going to ask her to be his wife. It would be, he was quite sure, an unforgettable day.

He would be right.

As Roumbi walked on, the village around him basked in lunchtime splendor, mustering what little bustle it had. Waiters scurried from table to table at Milord's and Madame Avril's restaurants, the smell of chicken and fish and bread wafting from their kitchens. Nearby, schoolchildren who'd gathered for phys-

ical examinations—Saturdays were school days in France—bub-
bled with chatter. Little girls with short-cropped hair played tag
at the *École des Filles*. In the marketplace, men waited for their
weekly tobacco ration and discussed the next day's football
match. Women shopped in the marketplace, then headed home
with their bargains and baguettes.

The village nestled on a gentle knoll, 150 miles southwest
of Paris. A church steeple rose above all else, a capital letter amid
an otherwise lower-case community. About 330 people lived
here, four times that many in the farmland beyond. They were
mainly Catholic, old-fashioned, and comfortable. Shops and
stone houses, some dating back to the fifteenth century, lined the
narrow main street that snaked through the middle of town, a
streetcar rail etched in its back. Beyond stretched a patchwork
quilt of rolling fields, neatly stitched together with hedgerows.

In a world at war, Oradour-sur-Glane was something of an
oasis. On weekends, clubs from the city of Limoges, fifteen miles
to the southeast, would come to spend the day on the banks of
the River Glane. People would swim and hold fishing contests as
the waters drifted lazily beneath the arched stone bridge that led
into town.

The Germans had occupied France now for four years,
since Hitler's panzer columns and goose-stepping soldiers bul-
lied into Paris in June 1940, unfurling their long, narrow Nazi
banners from the sides of buildings and sending millions of
refugees fleeing. But if Oradour-sur-Glane were technically part
of the Third Reich, it had long been treated with indifference by
the Germans, who, in their quest to conquer Europe, had more
pressing concerns. In fact, nobody had ever seen a German soldier here. The village lay as unfettered as an eddy-twirled leaf in
the River Glane.

Maurice Compain, a baker, rolled dough on a woodblock
table. Down the street, Clément Broussaudier leaned back in a

barber's chair for a haircut. And, at the southeastern entrance to town, two young women who had lunched together at the Hotel Milord—one a student from nearby Limoges—strolled across the arched stone bridge to part ways.

As the young woman from Oradour waved good-bye to her friend, she noticed something strange in the farmland to the southeast: dust rising from a road miles away. Not just the dust of a single vehicle, she realized, but dust from what looked to be many vehicles. The young woman turned and hurried to the village.

A SOLDIER'S BOOT kicked open the front door at the infants' school, freezing the children of Oradour-sur-Glane in fear. A Waffen-SS trooper brandished a gun. A panicked teacher told the children to lie facedown on the floor.

"*Raus!*" a soldier yelled, telling the children to get out. "*Raus!*" Vicious shouts peppered the village. Some children started crying. Some wet themselves.

Trucks and half-tracks rolled by, packed with soldiers dressed in green-and-brown camouflage smocks over field-gray uniforms. About 130 soldiers fanned out, yelling at the towns-people. "*Tout le monde sur la place!*" Everyone was to go to the marketplace. Shots rang out. Townspeople peered out their windows. What was happening?

The German detachment, the 3d company of the Waffen-SS's "Der Führer" Regiment, was part of the 2d Panzer Division known as "Das Reich." Its commander was Major Adolf Diekmann who, in the marketplace, demanded to see Mayor Jean Desourteaux. Speaking through an interpreter, he told Desourteaux that there was to be an identity check. All villagers were to assemble immediately.

Clément Broussaudier, seated in the barber's chair, heard

shots and hustled outside to get on his bicycle. A German soldier brusquely took it from him and said, in broken French, "You won't be needing it anymore."

Within an hour, hundreds of men, women, and children stood in the marketplace. Babies cried. Eyes darted right and left. A handful of German soldiers hastily mounted MG-42 machine guns on tripods. Others began separating the women and children from the men, forcing the former toward the nearby church at gunpoint. The sound of children's wooden shoes and the hobnailed soldiers' boots clattered from the cobblestones like mournful drums.

"*Singt,*" the soldiers suddenly shouted to the children in German. "*Singt!*" The children were frightened. But with guns pointed at them, the children of Oradour-sur-Glane began to sing, their mouths quivering. The women and children, hundreds of them, were pushed and prodded up the six steps and into the church. A frantic murmur raced through the throng.

Meanwhile, the men were divided into six groups, and herded into barns and garages around the marketplace. "Look out," whispered Joseph Bergmann, who knew German, to a friend, Marcel Darthout. "They are going to kill us!" Darthout did not believe him.

But in a horrifying burst of noise, machine-gun bullets riddled the Frenchmen in barns and garages now splattered red with blood. Men screamed, moaned, and cried out for loved ones. After the initial barrage, soldiers shot survivors in the head. Bodies were covered with straw and kindling, and barns and garages set afire. Soldiers swept through the village, torching houses and shops and shooting people forced out by the flames. Screams pierced the air. Machine guns rattled. A black-and-white dog named "Bobby" barked wildly along the River Glane. *Bang!* He barked no more.

At the church, soldiers burst in and fired machine guns at

the women and children, turning the stone sanctuary into a bloody swirl of pain and panic. Soldiers poured gasoline, stepped back, and lobbed hand grenades. Women and children writhed madly about and screamed in agony. They had become human torches.

When the madness finally stopped, 642 people, including 190 schoolchildren, lay dead or dying. Among them: Albert Roumbi and the young woman who was to be his wife. His daisies lay near his hand, trampled in the panic and soon to be scorched along with nearly everything else.

The German soldiers began torching every house and shop; more than three hundred structures were gutted to their foundations. The smell of burning flesh stained the air. Sewing machines, bicycles, toys, tables, dishes, wineglasses—the stuff of everyday life lay strewn in the rubble. All that was left were scarred foundations, chimneys, and a single house. No children sang in Oradour-sur-Glane.

Finally, near dark, the convoy of German soldiers loaded up and drove west out of town, the trucks and half-tracks full of loot they'd plundered from houses and shops. The SS men sat on the vehicles' benches, drinking, singing, and laughing. One played a festive German song on an accordion he'd pilfered from the debris.

It was time to leave. Time for more pressing business: to defend the Fatherland. Allied troops, the soldiers had heard, were pouring ashore about 250 miles northwest, in a place called Normandy.

CHAPTER 3

I heard him cry in sudden pain
I saw him fling his arms abroad,
And close his hands and jump—
Two paces forward—Then—
With sickening sound
He struck the ground.
A crimson liquid stain
Crept o'er the shadowed sand—
Then all was still again.
And dusk, and chill, and rain
Fell o'er us there . . .
      —FROM J. W. GOSLING'S *MY COMRADE*,
      FOUND IN FRANCES SLANGER'S CHAPBOOK

The Forty-fifth Field Hospital nurses had landed at a swath of beach labeled "Uncle Red," just off the inland village of La Madeleine. As Frances headed inland, the beach swirled with the activity of thousands of soldiers. The yawning mouths of the LCTs (Landing Craft, Tanks) disgorged men and equipment. Cranes unloaded pieces of artillery. GIs—"government-issue" soldiers, the tin-hatted grunts—hauled chests and crates, pulled the plastic sheaths off rifles, and ratcheted dry spark plugs into jeep motors. Ahead, trucks, tanks, and jeeps rolled inland through draws blown by navy demolition teams in the Germans' Atlantic Wall. It was 3:30 P.M., June 10.

Frances followed the others up the beach. It was flat, wide, and golden brown, giving way to sand dunes beyond that were sprinkled with beach grass and fronted by what looked to be pieces of driftwood. She stopped to hitch her musette bag onto her shoulder and suddenly caught a whiff of something that brought her back to her childhood in Lødz: the smell of death.

The pile of "driftwood" wasn't driftwood at all. It was the bodies of soldiers—not died-at-this-spot soldiers, but dead GIs who had been killed inland—a number were paratroopers from the 82nd and 101st Airborne Divisions—and been brought here for temporary burial. Frances stared at the carnage, soldiers wearing the face of death like the German soldiers she'd seen in World War I. Here and there, the wounded lay on stretchers or sat in the sand, some wrapped in bloodstained bandages, their heads bowed in their hands.

"Oh, my God," said Dottie Richter. This, she realized, wasn't Puerto Rico, where a soldier's worst enemy might be a blistering sunburn. Elizabeth Powers, her stomach still queasy from two days at sea, bent over. She retched.

Huddled together in the dunes, uniforms soaked to their skin, the nurses slowly began realizing the seriousness and scope of this operation. On a horizon now tinted with encroaching late-afternoon fog, the Channel was littered with ships big and small. Beneath wispy clouds, silver barrage balloons hovered above. What had been, in England, a neat, clean world of distinctive colors was now a collage of battleship grays and muted greens, blues, and browns. What had been, in England, thatched-roof cottages and rose-twined arbors and tidy vegetable gardens was now a muddle of the unnatural infringing on the natural: German hedgehogs, steel concoctions designed to rip the bottoms from landing craft, lay in piles like a child's jacks. Tanks, their treads clanking and squeaking, trampled through the beach grass that once arched in tints of green and gold. Half-submerged landing craft, like metal corpses, jutted from the shallows. Small waves rolled ashore. As the Forty-fifth Field Hospital waited for orders, light faded. And in sand scattered with cockle shells that now seemed utterly irrelevant to the world, the nurses' boot prints disappeared in the backwash.

CAPT. WILLIAM POE liked things to go his way. In England, when initially unable to secure billeting at a particular house to his liking, he had told the owner how disappointed he was that a descendant of "Edgar Allan himself"—*wink, wink*—might be turned away. Now, he strode purposefully down the beach, shaking his head. Things weren't going his way again. Not even ashore an hour and already there'd been another screwup—as if the ship positioning itself off Omaha hadn't been bad enough. Now, a ship carrying another field hospital, the Forty-second, had hit a mine and sunk; all personnel—seventy-four enlisted men and eight officers—had been saved but these units, and its nurses, weren't ashore yet.

Meanwhile, the Forty-second's surgeons, having arrived on another transport, were set up for business and had hundreds of waiting customers. It was the only functioning medical installation in the sector. The Forty-fifth's nurses were being called in as fill-ins. That would leave the Forty-fifth without nurses—but orders were orders. Poe huddled with other officers. Down the beach, the men of the Forty-fifth began arriving after coming across the Channel on what had been, in its prewar days, a British pleasure ship, the *Princess Maud*.

"Nurses, listen up!" yelled Poe, his voice only barely audible above the clamor. Frances and the others pressed forward.

"The Forty-second's docs have already set up shop but they've got no nurses. You're them. We leave in five."

The nurses were to hike to a village called Le Grand Chemin, about two miles inland. The rest of the Forty-fifth would head directly toward Ste.-Mère-Église, which had become, on D+1, the first town in France to be liberated.

"Let's make sure you're all here," said Poe, starting to read their names. "Belanger, Bowler, Cox . . ." Each nurse yelled a crisp "check" when her name was called. ". . . Fielden, Mahoney, Monroe, Montague, Morrison, Owen, Powers, Reynolds, Richter, Roe, Slanger . . ."

"Medic! Medic!" Down the dunes from Frances and the other nurses, Capt. Joseph Shoham of the Forty-fifth Field Hospital heard the cry from somewhere up ahead. He turned to see a medic emerge from a foxhole to answer the call for help. *Phhht.* The bullet hit him just above the eye. A spurt of blood misted the twilight air. It was the first time Shoham had ever seen a man die. Within five minutes he'd see all sorts of death, including a pile of Germans, most of whom looked too young to shave. Shoham noticed rings on some of their fingers. He was surprised the bands hadn't been taken as souvenirs by American GIs.

He moved forward with the others. The hiss of an incoming shell filled the air. "G'down!" someone yelled. "And watch for mines!" In some areas, the Germans had sown them like crop seed.

Streams of jeeps, trucks, half-tracks, tanks, and ambulances headed inland on exits punched through the dunes. In the gathering twilight, the column rolled past fields purposely flooded by the Germans and littered with American paratroopers who'd drowned in the early morning darkness of D-Day, some still wrapped like mummies in their parachutes. Wooden stakes—"Rommel's asparagus"—angled in the ground, where they'd been rammed by the Germans to thwart the landing of gliders and paratroopers. Shoham heard the *crack, crack, crack* of an M-1. He turned. Not far away, GIs were shooting German POWs at point-blank range. He swallowed hard, turned, and moved on.

"Move along now!" officers barked. "Move along!"

Capt. Fred Michalove, a former newspaper reporter and now the chief administrative officer of Frances's Second Platoon, came around a curve in the road and suddenly stopped, so stunned was he at the sight: Paratroopers—guys who'd once hoisted beers across from him at the same Pump Tavern in Fayetteville, North Carolina—hung from trees, their chutes having gotten hung up in the branches. The Germans had used the soldiers for target practice; some looked like butcher-shop carcasses hanging in a walk-in freezer. Michalove stopped. He wanted to cut them down, to save these dead soldiers from further humiliation, but the mass of men and machines surged forward and he with it.

The push inland continued, through breaks in lines of barbed wire, past farmhouses in rubble, and around apple orchards charred by bombs. At the end of the snaking column of troops and vehicles, Capt. Emanuel D. Berson, a Forty-fifth dental officer, suddenly realized he'd left his gas mask on the beach. He left the formation to go back and get it, having to skirt the main road to avoid the flow of oncoming troops. *Blam!* Sand exploded into the sky. Berson was blown sideways. Shrapnel from a *Luftwaffe* bomb tore into his stomach. It didn't kill him, but it shredded his colon so badly that doctors would later have to remove a foot of it. Those in the Forty-fifth never saw the man again.

NOTHING IN WAR triggers fleeting introspection like the sight and smell of the dead, because among the swirling emotions rises an unavoidable truth: *If he can die here and now, so can I.*

"If you say you're not scared, you'll be a cocky fool,"
Frances had read in her *Army Life* manual. "Don't let anyone tell
you you're a coward if you admit being scared. Fear, before
you're actually in the battle, is a normal emotional reaction. It's
the last step of preparing . . ."

Frances trudged on with the other nurses, looking at the
ruins of war and the men who'd already died in it. Tanks smoked,
their charred victims littered in all sorts of contortions of death.
Flies toyed with the bloated bodies of soldiers and cows. A lone
boot lay here, a severed hand there. Chaplains held impromptu
services for the dead, surrounded by haggard soldiers holding
rifles and bowing their heads. For some who'd already given
their lives in the first four days in France, there wasn't even time
for that. Their bodies were buried with bulldozers.

For years, Frances had dared to look the world straight in
the eye—at its utter worst. She had clipped and saved magazine
and newspaper articles about the atrocities in Eastern Europe.
"Even in death," she had written after a young mother had died
at Boston City Hospital, "I cannot help but think how much
more fortunate she is than millions of other human beings elsewhere." Now, Frances was in that "elsewhere."

When enlisting, she had filled out her last will and testament, a surprisingly simple one-sentence statement that asked
her to name her beneficiary. (She chose her parents.) She understood what it meant when told to choose someone to notify "in
case of emergency." (She chose her sister.) But if landing at
Normandy hammered home the reality of death, a worse fear
clung to Frances with the chill of her wet fatigues: the fear of
failure. To die was inevitable, Frances Slanger had long believed.
To die in vain—for no purpose at all—was not.

An officer of the Forty-second Field Hospital met the
nurses and led them toward Le Grand Chemin, just northwest of
Ste.-Marie-du-Mont. The nurses trudged on, among them

Frances, weighed down not only by heavy, wet clothes and gear, but an encroaching fear. Nearly drowning while coming ashore had diluted what little confidence she'd had. The sight of the wounded and the dead had deepened the fear of failure within. But ready or not, it was time. Time to channel her poetic patriotism into action. Time, finally, to go to war.

THE NUDGE from her father came early, long before morning light had found its way into her family's third-floor flat in Boston's South End. *Frances, s'iz tzite ooftzeshtain* came the Yiddish whisper. Time to wake up. Time to go sell the fruit. Time to go to work.

The Slangers lived in a three-decker row house that faced north on Oneida Street, a quarter-mile long artery that linked Harrison Avenue and Albany Street. Sixty such row houses were packed together, thirty on each side, like two lines of dominoes placed on end. Half a mile away, from the east, rumbled cars from the Boston & Albany Railroad Company's terminal. Two blocks away, from the west, clacked the Boston Elevated Railway. Nearly all such flats were filled with Jewish immigrants who had begun escaping Eastern Europe beginning with the Russian *pogroms* in 1881, survivors welcomed by relatives as if shipwrecked sailors clinging to the same life raft. Soon after arriving in 1920, Regina and her two daughters, Chaja and Freidel, had had their names changed. Regina became Eva. Chaja became Sarah, though she was called Sally. And Freidel became Frances.

Now, in the rare quiet of morning, Frances left with her father. It was April 1926, spring by the calendar, winter by the weather. Spots of ice made the cobblestones slippery, all beneath a 5 A.M. sky as dark as carbon paper. It was a Thursday, reason to thank God, Frances's father would often tell her: Tomorrow would be the Sabbath and so today the fruit would sell fast. Her father coughed a cough that twelve-year-old Frances knew well by now. He was a small man, five-foot-three with brown eyes, brown hair, a round face, cursive lips, and jug ears. He was known as one of the hardest-working fruit peddlers around. He wore glasses, and on mornings like this, fingerless woolen gloves. Frances already had on her mittens. After seven years in Poland and nearly six in Boston, she understood cold.

As father and daughter walked the streets toward the stables, near the Washington/Dover street area, David lit the first of many cigarettes he would smoke on this day. At the stables, a brick building resembling a firehouse, Frances watched as he hitched the horse to a cart that had wood-spoked wheels taller than she. He helped her up, climbed on himself, then twitched the reins and guided the horse a couple of miles east, to a market in South Boston, the city's Irish enclave. Father and daughter sat next to each other, but always with distance between. In the eyes of Frances, her father was a gentle man. He had allowed her to have a dog, Yip-Yip, a German shepherd. And as he dealt with customers, she learned how to deal with people, too. But he was a distant man, a man she hadn't even seen until she was seven years old and, at times, still seemed far away.

In the South End, Frances came to be known as the fruit peddler's daughter, even if she felt more like Eva's daughter, the daughter of the woman who had gotten her through a war, across an ocean, and beyond Ellis Island. Eva Slanger had premature gray hair that was cut short and pulled back. Her face, behind round-rimmed glasses, was creased deeply with worry lines that she nurtured daily. She was the classic Jewish *baleboste*—household manager—whose love of family pulsed through the clacking of her sewing machine, through the back-and-forth whoosh of a broom, and through fingers kneading dough for Sabbath bread.

Smaller than David by half a head, she was built like a fire hydrant. Smiles came hard for Eva Slanger. But in the eyes of Frances, her mother was a pillar of strength, a comforter, "more loving than others I see," she once wrote in a poem. "Noble of mind . . . a teacher of right from wrong." In her mother, Frances saw a hard-crusted, softhearted woman who had all but willed herself, and her two girls, to survive. In Lødz, the three had felt the gnaw of hunger and smelled the bloated bodies of the dead and heard the moans of diseased children after typhoid swept through the city.

The dangers of Boston were mild by comparison. On mornings like these, when the Irish boys—the smart-aleck *shgotzim*, her father called them—were still in bed, this area would not scare her. In the afternoon, when she and her father returned for more fruit, it would. She had seen what the boys sometimes did: tipping over the carts of the Jewish peddlers, grabbing armloads of fruit, and saying "thanks" with a well-placed tomato to the man's chest or face, laughing as they fled. But it was not like the German soldiers in Lødz, who were known to do far worse.

Finally, with the cart loaded for the day, Frances and her father headed back to the South End to begin the route. A bleak morning sun bled through hazy clouds to the east, over the Atlantic Ocean—perhaps poetic fodder for Frances, the young writer.

"*Oon frishe frucht!*" her father yelled. "*Eplin, bahren, floimen, orahnges, pine'eplin, vassermelon!*" His Yiddish cries mixed with the chants of the other Jewish peddlers to comprise a spirited and predictable chorus. Across Harrison Avenue, the voice of another fruit peddler, Morris Zola, added to the Yiddish choir. Zola, a Russian Jew, worked the west side of Harrison, David Slanger the east. They were competitors but helped one another. *You're out of cherries, my friend? I give you cherries. Why? Because someday I will be out of cherries.*

Because he sold bootleg booze on the side during these Prohibition years, Morris Zola was able to afford the first telephone on the block. He had a son, Milton, who was eight years younger than Frances. She was like a big sister to him. They knew each other well enough to know each other's Yiddish names: his was *"Motle,"* hers *"Faigie."* They lived four blocks apart. The Zolas lived on Florence Street. But the two saw each other most often from the backs of horse-drawn wagons as the South End came to life each morning, a gritty urban haven for Jews who had known far worse.

The smell of fresh herring, coal-fed fires, and Old World cooking blended with horse manure and the occasional waft of raw sewage that emptied into the Fort Point Channel beyond the coal and lumber yards, just east of the Slanger flat. It was more ghetto than town, an urbanized American *shtetl*, safe from the hounding of the South Boston hoodlums and far from the upturned noses of Beacon Hill's elite.

Owners of the South End's ramshackle stores and kosher markets started stacking their sidewalk displays with pumpernickel bread, bagels, sausages, and skinned chickens. Laundry hung on lines from one tenement window to the next, fluttering in the same breeze that bent the factory smoke beyond. Horses clomped down the streets, making way for the burnt-orange trolleys and the occasional hand-cranked Model T—all of it slightly blurry for a little girl whose vision was poor.

"Lebediker fisch, weiber, lebediker fisch!" Frances heard the fish peddler yell.

The Jewish women leaned out their windows and yelled orders to David. He weighed the fruit, placed it in a paper sack, marked the price on the bag, and Frances ran to deliver it. Then she returned, sometimes out of breath, with the coins.

By now, most of the more successful Jews in Boston, including the German Jews who looked decidedly down on the

Polish Jews—"greenhorns"—had moved farther south to Roxbury and Dorchester, places where some streets had gas lamps lit by lamplighters on stilts. Oneida Street wasn't among them; Frances's father made $5 to $10 per day, meaning it took about a week to earn the monthly rent.

Ah, but for this, you thanked God, her father said. Milton Zola's father said the same thing. Mr. Zola often reminded Milton that America's streets were paved with gold. "But, Papa," his son said one morning as they sat, side by side, on their horse-drawn wagon, "the streets—they are not gold."

"Don't you understand, my son?" Mr. Zola said. "Your *freedom* is your gold. You don't have to worry that someone is going to kill you, that a Christian is going to kill you, that the Russians are going to kill you. You don't have to worry about moving from one town to the other. You can sell your cherries and your apples. You can dig a ditch. *This* is your freedom."

This, too, is what Frances's father taught her: that despite the cold winter months when profits froze along with the ponds, despite the heat of summer when the Slangers' top-floor apartment warmed like an oven, despite $3 days, and the South Boston toughs, this was your freedom. Realize it. Cherish it. Defend it.

As THE YEARS PASSED, Frances carved out a place to be alone, a hideaway from the world: up on the roof, above the family's South End flat. How *ever* could she hope to become an internationally known author down below in the apartment? Did Massachusetts authors like Henry Thoreau or Louisa May Alcott spin their prose while packed into an oversized cracker box with three other people—one a boy-blinded sister? With Yiddish chatter? With a father's annoying cough?

Of course not. Nor did Beethoven, she had read in a magazine article that she'd glued into her chapbook. His ideas "came best in the open air" and he "once wrote an oratorio" while "sitting in the fork of a favorite lime tree in the Schoenbrunn Gardens." Somehow, amid the oppressive brick and stone of the South End, Frances needed her own Schoenbrunn Gardens. And she found them in her perch on the roof, even if her hideaway's entire plant life consisted of a single potted fern.

The spot lacked the solitude of Cape Cod and New Hampshire's Lake Nubanusit, where, thanks to relatives with far more money than her family had, Frances had visited in summers past. But it was at least a place to be alone. Wooden decking covered the flat roof. A fence made of roughhewn 2 x 10s guarded the edges. Frances draped a plaid blanket over the fence to give the rooftop nook a semblance of privacy and to lessen the chances that the stickball boys on Oneida Street would chortle "bookworm" chants her way. The fern and an old rug added ambience and gave Yip-Yip, her German shepherd, a soft place to curl up. At times, she would bring a caged parakeet with her on the roof. The setup wasn't exactly Beethoven with his sketch pad "out roaming the fields, singing, roaring, humming, gesticulating and scribbling." But it would do for now.

Frances had two childhood dreams; one was to be a writer. It was here, on the roof, where she fell in love with words, reading them and writing them. Words could make her laugh, cry, and wonder. They could seal in her memory a sunrise above the Fort Point Channel. They could be portals to make-believe worlds, places where she could sail first-class, not steerage. And they could offer hope.

She wrote of her mother, of freedom, of willing one's self to never give up, and of nature, the latter inspired largely by summer trips to Cape Cod. She wrote a fairy tale, "The Queen of Hate and Prince Sweetface," in which a hateful queen learns to love after a young prince plants a row of forget-me-nots and melts the hate in the queen's heart. In an odd twist for a Jewish girl, she even created, and sent out, her own Christmas cards.

Everywhere she looked she found something to appreciate, something to ponder, something to wonder about. In one poem she wrote:

> Wouldn't you all like to know,
> Why rivers turn and oceans flow?
> Where Jack and Jill fell off the hill,
> And why the winds can be so still?
>
> Why are all the leaves so green?
> Why, at night, is nothing seen?
> What makes night and what makes day,
> Can you tell me please, I pray?

With the persistence of Boston's winter snows, her teachers at Abraham Lincoln Intermediate School reminded the class that good readers make good writers. So Frances became a serious reader, difficult because she had poor eyesight. She often took a streetcar to the new South End branch of the Boston Public Library that had opened in 1923. She learned to type. She made bookmarks with inspirational quotes by some of her favorite authors: Shakespeare. Emerson. Milton. She wrote out notes on improving her poetry, on the use of figures of speech, on grammar symbols. She typed out some of her favorite poems, including John Masefield's "Sea Fever" and John McCrae's World War I epic, "In Flanders Fields."

Had she been a Jewish boy, her parents might have encouraged such an interest. Even if they couldn't read what she'd written, they might have at least ascribed means-to-an-end value to her silly stories and poems—good training for the days when a son might go off to Harvard College and make the family proud.

Jewish males won considerable distinction at the prestigious Boston Public Latin School, which sent more students to Harvard than any public school in the nation. And behind them stood families who sacrificed so their sons might soar.

Behind Jewish daughters, meanwhile, stood matchmaking mothers. Women in America may have won the vote in 1920 and been awash in new privileges, but Jewish parents were still more interested in their daughters landing successful men. Most Jewish girls weren't encouraged to *become* anything; instead, they were expected to help their parents, to bake and scrub, and to prepare for the Jewish holidays.

Teachers, then, became gods of approval. Once, a teacher at Abraham Lincoln swept down the classroom rows, passing out corrected writing papers. Frances, nearly cowering in her chair, waited anxiously. Finally, the teacher handed Frances's assignment back to her. The girl's eyes raced to the end, to where perhaps the teacher had written remarks that could make her believe anything—that someday, for example, she might write words that would inspire people near and far. Instead, the teacher wrote: "You must be Polish. Brush up on your grammar."

The words stung. But Frances hung on to whatever thread of hope she had. "When lights are dim and things look dark," she wrote, "don't fail to climb to a nobler mark. Carry on!"

It was an almost instinctive optimism, a will to overcome that was rooted deep in the winters of Lødz. That's how life worked. She'd seen it. Like your mother, you pumped the wooden handle until realizing no water was going to come out; the pipes were frozen. Then you began to melt snow.

By AGE FIFTEEN, having grown out her hair and begun wearing long dresses that cut against the grain of the short-skirt twenties,

Frances looked every bit the struggling bohemian writer that she fashioned herself to be. "This is an original story," she once wrote atop a piece of work, as if some magazine editor might believe it were so good she'd copied something from, say, Edna St. Vincent Millay.

Her aspirations as a writer exceeded her skills, fueling all sorts of hopes and dreams. She would leave the grimy confines of Boston and live in the woods like Henry David Thoreau had, writing and watching the nuances of nature change from season to season. ("How I wish I were now in Cape Cod/Where the tree tops gently seem to nod/Where the . . . breezes softly blow/Where the larkspur and snapdragon grow. . . .") She would be the next Millay, the poet of bohemian rebellion who'd won a Pulitzer Prize at age thirty. She would prove to herself and the world that if you wanted something badly enough—if you dared to make a difference—you could find that something. You could make a difference.

The spirit of her writing, however, was richer than the quality of her writing. In one poem, she wrote: "Let's drink to them who say 'I will'/For they shall reach the top of the hill." With English coming to her late, grammar and spelling were never her strengths. But her pieces gurgled with passion, optimism, and innocence. "Fears and sorrows will diminish fast,/All your troubles will be of the past;/Look to the future, face the sun;/For indeed your life has just begun."

In a world of flappers, Frances maintained a certain frumpiness—the "author's look"—except when at school, where uniforms were required. At Lincoln Intermediate School, which stood on Tremont Street and required a mile's walk from her home, Frances wore a white, short-sleeved blouse with a navy blue scarf pulled through a wooden ring; a blue skirt that fell just below the knees; blue tights; and white, ankle-high shoes. Frances's teachers were almost all Irish Catholic, her classmates

Irish and seemingly everything else. The South End had the largest number of blacks in Boston. Her class was comprised of Italians, Germans, Greeks, Asians, Indians, and plenty of Eastern Europeans like herself. In this ethnic collage, her classmates were kids named Rose Aryvosios, Angelino Di Di, Ida Dross, Harry Kostasky, Beatrice Spegel, and Morris Yanoff, whose family was close friends with hers. For the most part, ghetto kids. South End kids. And some of them quietly burdened kids.

The Eastern European Jews, in particular, found themselves living in two worlds. Yiddish was spoken at home, English in the classroom. After school, Frances would arrive home, leaving her English at the front door as if it were an umbrella to be stowed, having already served its purpose. The next morning, she was off to school, where even having a lunch wrapped in a Yiddish newspaper could cause a teacher's eyes to roll.

Unlike her parents, who learned little more than rudimentary English, Frances had picked up the new language quickly. She carried messages from her parents to doctors, landlords, and shopkeepers. One day, after telephones had become widely available in the twenties, a man from the local telephone company showed up at Frances's Lincoln School. There, in the brick building, he met with the scores of immigrant children for one purpose: to explain how the new device worked, so they, in turn, could explain to their parents how it worked. "Go-betweens," they were called—immigrant children who, in some ways, took on dual roles: adult and child. It was a role Frances would come to know well. At times, too well.

On the roof, she would sit and listen to the sounds of the day fading—the bark of a dog, the *clack-clack-de-clack-clack* of the Boston & Albany cars, and the marital shouting matches in any of a dozen flats within earshot, perhaps the one right beneath her. It couldn't have been easy for David and Eva, this adjustment to America—and to each other. Seven years before, when they had reunited in America, each was grappling with new roles, new rules, and seven years of missing time. David expected Eva to embrace America's ways as if it meant nothing more than a change of clothes, not easy for a woman rooted in the Old Country. Eva expected David to be unchanged from the man who had left Lødz in 1913, equally hard for a man who'd washed his hands of the Old Country.

Their marriage, like most turn-of-the-century unions in Poland, had sprung from the mind of a matchmaker, not their desire for each other. And though they may well have grown to love each other deeply, they also may have been as distant as passengers in first-class are from those in steerage. As Frances grew up, her night-sky dreams brought visions that took her beyond her parents, beyond the cold, confining ways of the city, beyond anything she'd ever known. In a poem called "Freedom" she wrote:

> I wish I were away,
> Where carefree gypsies stay,
> Where little brooklets play.
> Away from city noise,
> And rough and careless boys,
> And ugly human toys . . .
> To eat when e'r I please,
> To lie beneath the trees,
> And welcome every breeze . . .

In time, her freedom would come, though not in the idyllic way her poetry suggested.

CHAPTER 4

You cannot dream yourself into a character—you must hammer and forge yourself one.

—ANONYMOUS,
FOUND IN FRANCES SLANGER'S CHAPBOOK

Night fell on Normandy, not that anybody much noticed. The eighteen nurses of the Forty-fifth Field Hospital neared Le Grand Chemin with senses too overloaded by everything else. German and American planes rumbled overhead. Antiaircraft fire lit up the night sky like crazed fireworks. On the ground, words had to be shouted over the thunder of war. *Whump-whump-whump-whump* . . .

Onward the nurses trudged, wet clothes matted to their bodies. Too-large boots squished with salt water. Foot blisters formed, then popped and chaffed. The brackish smell of sea and diesel gave way to plain diesel, with occasional whiffs of dead bodies that Graves Registration hadn't gotten to. Finally, in the murky darkness, the nurses made out the vague outline of what appeared to be a field hospital tent. Inside, flashlight beams gyrated like fireflies with the silhouetted comings and goings of doctors and medics. The nurses came to a halt. A thirtyish man in scrubs, blood up to his elbows and surgical mask around his neck, poked his head out the flap of the tent and swept a flashlight beam across the newcomers.

"My God," he said, "nurses!"

He was a doctor from the Third Auxiliary surgical unit that was supporting the Forty-second Field Hospital. The unit had erected tents in a pasture just north of Le Grand Chemin; at this point, it was the only medical facility operating in the sector.

"Let's go, girls!" said Captain Hay, the Forty-fifth's leader.

The operating room was comprised of four stretchers laid across footlockers. With no generators on hand yet to supply light, surgeries were being done by flashlight. Most of the Forty-second's supplies hadn't made it; some never would, resting, as they were, on the bottom of the English Channel in the ship that had struck a mine. The only thing the Forty-second had in abundance was patients. The waiting room was literally being measured by the truckload—seventeen at one point. Some soldiers had been waiting two days for medical attention. Others could wait no longer. They wouldn't be attended to by nurses or doctors, but by Graves Registration soldiers, some of whom had already found the only way to do their grisly job was to get drunk and stay drunk.

Frances Slanger peered into the tent. Stale light shone from a few hanging lanterns, casting shadows on the cotton-duck walls and bringing the nurses face-to-face with the reason they were here: tired, dirty, bloody soldiers, some draped for surgery, others waiting their turn. The GIs' eyes drooped with desperation, some with shame. It was as if the soldiers wanted attention but didn't believe they deserved it, as if they somehow felt guilty for dragging the innocent into what, in only four days, had already become a horrific mess. Soft moans rose here and there, the audio equal of sea chop. The arm of a just-arrived GI dangled by a lone tendon. The smell of gangrene hung like a putrid fog.

Frances Slanger had never seen, heard, or smelled anything like it. She hesitated, frozen by the scene before her. She stared for a moment. Then she pitched her musette bag aside and, along with the others, grabbed a cloth surgical gown.

"Where," she said, "can we get flashlights?"

As part of the only medical hospital in the area—and the first nurses to actually care for D-Day wounded—the Forty-fifth Field Hospital nurses were soon awash in the blood of the living, the dead, and those hanging perilously in between. Red stained the cloth surgical gowns that once were white, all colors muted in the cave-like tents. The blood exuded a strong, musky smell with a touch of metallic—something not easily forgotten, like the fear in a wounded soldier's eyes. Or like triage.

With canvas stretchers lined up in open fields, doctors from the Third Auxiliary and Forty-Second units went from soldier to soldier, deciding who could wait and who could not; by 10 P.M., 300 patients had been admitted. Some soldiers had their field dressings checked and were given only essential treatment. Then they were fed, given a hot drink, and transferred to the 261st Engineers Medical Battalion back on the beach; from there, they'd be shipped back to England.

If a soldier wasn't already dead, he desperately needed surgery—often two days ago. Still others, though composed, were battling wounds that drew no blood, but were deep nevertheless: battle fatigue. The thousand-yard stare. Slack lips. A sleepwalker's stance. Many had been fighting nonstop for four days. They hadn't slept. They'd seen buddies killed in all sorts of ways, sometimes as innocently as reaching for a souvenir Luger or belt buckle on a dead German—only to find the body had been booby-trapped. Cigarettes jiggled in the fingers of the dazed Americans, the ashes growing long. When Frances bent over such soldiers outside the tent, their eyes looked right through her, to a darkness ablaze with gunfire.

Shortly after 10 P.M., German planes bombed and strafed an area so close to the medical tents that surgeons scrambled for their helmets and some of the wounded were dragged into fox-holes. The insides of the tents flickered dark and light as if caught in a thunderstorm. Cannons flashed and roared.

Frances ripped open sulfanilamide and sulfathiazole pack-ets and poured the infection-fighting powder on wounds, the likes of which she'd never seen before. She helped doctors stop bleeders that burbled like underground springs. She searched, sometimes in vain, for blankets, bandages, or other supplies lost in the chaos. She lit soldiers' cigarettes. And she tried to smile at the wounded as if to say everything was going to be all right.

"Mama . . . Mama," said a soldier whose head was wrapped like a mummy's. Captain Hay, Frances realized, had been right in what she'd told the nurses in a training session at Fort Bragg: Soldiers didn't cry out for wives or girlfriends or even God. They almost always cried out for their mothers.

A chaplain, splattered with blood and fueled by something beyond his own strength, whispered a prayer in the left ear of a man who no longer had a right. ". . . Yea, though I walk though the valley of the shadow of death, I will fear no evil, for Thou *art* with me. . . ."

"Damn it, we lost him," muttered a nearby surgeon about another patient.

As the night deepened, enlisted men outside the tents dug foxholes. Beyond, others dug graves. Inside, the surgical battle continued. In two hours, Frances had already seen more death and misery than in her seven years at Boston City Hospital. Like the others, she was exhausted, but kept going. Who knows what sustained her: perhaps some "carry-on-despite-the-odds" poem she'd written on her apartment roof in Boston. Some quick prayer whispered with urgency while she fumbled around in a trunk for more bandages. Some subconscious image of helpless German soldiers on a horse cart in Lødz. Perhaps a touch of all, but no force so strong as simply the adrenaline-pulsed mandate to do her job as a nurse, whether it be while standing on the waxed linoleum at Boston City or in the blood-tinged fields of Normandy.

The nurses didn't eat a thing until 11 P.M., and then only C-rations. They went to the bathroom in foot-wide slit trenches: straddle and squat. They had been awake now for almost twenty-four hours, having spent nearly two hours getting to shore, another couple shivering on the beach, and an hour hiking. Now, they were assisting doctors they'd never met, patching wounds like they'd never seen for soldiers they'd never forget.

Sallylou, just after helping a doctor amputate a soldier's leg—and wiping down the saw with alcohol—finally was given her first break. She went outside into the darkness and leaned against the rise of a hedgerow. Her head pounded with the roar of planes and bombs and antiaircraft artillery fire. Her fatigues were wet with blood, her injured foot aching all the more because of the hike and having not sat down for hours.

Whatever she had expected of France, this wasn't it. Back home, nursing had had a certain romance to it. When she had graduated from St. Luke's Hospital's program in Racine, Wisconsin, each nurse carried a "Florence Nightingale lamp," symbolic of the much-revered British nurse who had cared for the wounded soldiers during the Crimean War.

Now, eyes heavy, Sallylou watched as flashlight beams inside the tents darted here and there amid assembly-line surgeries.

When Sallylou had trained at Camp Ellis in Illinois, the *Chicago Tribune* published a photo package to show what the Army Nurse Corps was supposedly all about. The photos, provided by the army, were of four nurses trying on gas masks with the levity of a pajama party; a group of smiling nurses curling their eyelashes, combing their hair, and drinking Coca-Cola; and nurses assisting in a "surgery," their surgical gowns white as country snow.

Nothing was white in Normandy. On the ground, brown, green, and blood-red were the colors of note, all shrouded in a surreal darkness streaked with multicolor tracers. Beneath the glow of such tracers and the throb of planes, another nurse came out of the tent, twisting her head right and left to get out the kinks. It was Frances Slanger, who paused when she saw the dim outline of a fellow nurse on the ground.

"That you, Sallylou?" she said over the noise.

"What's left of me," said Cummings.

Inside the tent, a soldier groaned. "Nobody expected this," said Frances.

Sallylou took a swig of water from a canteen. "Feel like a short-order cook on half-off night," she said, then handed the canteen to Frances. "What are we doing here, Slanger?"

THE FIST caught Milton Zola in the corner of the mouth with the sound of a splattered tomato. He was eight at the time and had been standing on Blue Hill Avenue, selling copies of the Boston *Record-American*, when the kid attacked. His lip bleeding, his jaw numb, his eyes tearing, Milton chased the boy into St. Matthew's Catholic Church, where a priest apprehended the young thug.

Such was life for a "Jew boy," as the attackers called Zola and his friends. They felt like hunted animals, fighting their way to and from school because they had the blood of a Jew. "He's a *Hebe!*" someone would sneer, and the fists would flail. Some who witnessed such beatings walked away. Some grew angry but didn't act, and some rolled up their sleeves to exact revenge.

A young Frances Slanger reacted differently. She'd ignore the assailant. Instead, she'd go to the boy who'd been beaten. She'd want to stop the bleeding, to comfort him. In fact, as she neared her high school years, Frances nurtured a small second dream. Beyond wanting to be a writer, she also wanted to be a nurse.

She tried on the idea cautiously, as if it were a new dress that seemed finer than anything she might deserve. And yet she found it a perfect fit. "I want to serve they who are less fortunate than I," she wrote, her words—as was often the case—more passionate than grammatically correct. "I have always loved to comfort those who were sick." This is how she would become, in the Jewish faith, a *mensch*, an ideal, ethical human being. A complete person.

For a Jewish girl, however, these were forbidden waters. She was expected to help her mother take care of the family, perhaps picking up some factory work on the side, then marry a Jewish man, preferably a doctor or lawyer or business owner. If the family had money, such a girl might find a way to escape the traditional expectations. But for the daughter of a fruit peddler to become a nurse was as ludicrous as her father selling fresh strawberries in January.

"It's *not* for a Jewish girl!" Such was a common refrain among Jewish parents whose daughters raised the possibility. Nursing was seen by many as a "Christian calling." It was for the pork-eaters. Hospitals didn't even offer kosher food. But by age fourteen—half her life now having been spent in America—Frances continued on her quiet quest. *Hadn't that English woman, Florence Nightingale, become a nurse against her parents' wishes?*

Beyond comforting the occasional beat-up boy, Frances found other outlets for her desire to be a nurse. The Yanoffs down the street had two boys who were disabled: Samuel, seven years younger than Frances, had polio, and Henry, eleven years younger, had cerebral palsy. Frances would routinely take them for walks—Samuel was in a wheelchair—and sometimes to a movie at the nearby Morton Theater. "Someday," she proudly told Joseph Yanoff, one of eleven brothers and eight years her junior, "I'm going to be a nurse."

She had a bent for taking care of people. She spent a summer at Cape Cod babysitting a blond-haired girl about half her age. She waited tables at resorts. And she grew to liking the idea of being a nurse. One evening at dinner, seemingly out of nowhere, Frances mentioned that idea to her parents. David and Eva looked at each other. Frances's heart surged with hope; one nod of approval from her parents and she could soar! Her parents looked back at Frances. Then they broke out in laughter, scoffing at the idea. Why, they wondered, couldn't she be more like Sally? Why, when she came of age, couldn't she find *ahn oisgetzaichenter yunger mah*—a prized young man? Frances's head bent down. She knew she could never measure up to Sally, nor did she want to try. They were both immigrant girls, sisters with the same last names; beyond that, the two had little in common.

Sally was nearly seven years older than Frances so the two shared little in the way of common interests or challenges. Sally was, at least in her own eyes, a rising flapper-in-waiting, a sophisticate. Frances was one of the only girls in her class to wear glasses—she'd finally gotten them, probably at the insistence of teachers. Her nickname was "Bud."

Sylvia Fine, a cousin of the girls from New Jersey, would come for a visit and find Sally rolling on the latest shade of lipstick in front of her mother's mirror. Frances, meanwhile, would be curled up on the roof with a book. Serious. Introspective. An unusual girl, Sylvia thought, as if living in another world than most. And yet intriguing for that very reason.

Sally and her friends dipped deeply into an increasingly anything-goes America during the twenties that all but ignored the hard-fought gains of their feminist elders: skirts were up, morals down, bobbed hair in, responsibility out. At the "talkies," Sally and her friends flirted with boys in the back rows of the Morton Theater. In the winter, they ice-skated at Roxbury's Franklin Park after the Parks Department flooded it and

Boston's winter froze it. Sally developed a shine for a young Jewish man named James Sidman.

Frances, meanwhile, dedicated herself to the carrying out of the Ten Commandments that she'd learned in three years of Hebrew school and that were posted in the Beth Han Hagodol Synagogue to which the family belonged. She culled and clipped inspirational writings from magazines for her chapbook. She immersed herself in Elbert Hubbard's "doing of the right thing," going so far as to write out the ethics of joke-telling. ("Laugh *with* people, not *at* people . . . Avoid coarseness and vulgarity.") She wrote poems honoring "those who say 'I will'/For they will reach the top of the hill." And she fell in love with the natural world that was so hard to find in the gritty South End. Inspired by summer trips to Cape Cod and Flying Loon Farm near Lake Nubanusit in New Hampshire, she glorified nature in verse. She walked in the rain—"it takes away the pain."

Sally liked jazz; it helped her escape life's drudgery. Frances liked classical music; it inspired "courage and thoughts of hope," she once wrote. "Magic into you comes stealing/All your thoughts and all your feelings." Sally danced; Frances dreamed. Not that Frances, on occasion, wasn't envious of her sister's free-wheeling ways. In one short story, she wrote of a character, Joan, who "[looked] longingly at her sister's new nile green evening gown" and begged her sibling to let her wear it to the country club dance Saturday night. Her sister said no. "Joan sat down at the table and buried her head in her arms," Frances wrote. "Agonized sobs shook her small, graceful body. . . ."

Despite her occasional forays into such fantasy, though, Frances stayed clear of what she saw as her sister's more trifling ways, and fixed her eyes somewhere beyond the "city noise." On her bedroom wall hung a picture of a beautiful nurse, standing madonna-like in some European villa, a white cape wrapped around her shoulders, a pitcher of water in her hands—water awaiting the parched lips of a patient.

• • •

IN NORMANDY, Frances Slanger tipped the mouth of a canteen to a soldier's lips. Her sleeves were rolled up, her olive-green shirt sticky from sweat and the salty residue of the English Channel. Splotches of blood smeared her once-neat uniform, making it look like the paint smock of a child with a penchant for crimson. She wiped her brow with her forearm, every split-second of respite doused by a doctor needing this or another nurse needing that.

In tents whose stifling air warmed with each passing hour, the nurses' first night blended unceremoniously into their first full day. The bone-weary pace continued. By 6 A.M. on June 11, the surgical backlog was 114 cases long. Frances noticed Dottie Richter looking at her hands: They were bleeding, having been rubbed raw by the scissors used to cut uniforms off soldiers.

"I keep losing mine," said Frances.

"Try this," said Dottie, showing how she'd tied a bandage to the scissors and kept them like a pocket watch.

"Nurse, help me plug this leak, now!" said a panicked surgeon, asking Frances for a task she'd never done. She plugged the artery, once she'd found it amid the wet, red gristle.

"Need fresh batteries!" yelled a doctor behind her, his "surgical light" going dim.

Gradually, a few nurses—backs aching, minds numb—were allowed to get some food and sleep, heading for foxholes or burrowing into hedgerows, using their inflated life belts for pillows. There'd been no time to put up tents. And their bedrolls had not yet reached them, apparently still on the beach or wrongly routed to Ste.-Mère-Église with the men's gear.

At nightfall at the end of the Forty-fifth's first full day in Normandy, someone put two cans of C-rations in Sallylou Cummings's hands and told her to get some shut-eye. She found a blanket, lay her head on a life belt and fell fast asleep, the cans still in her hands. Frances was nowhere to be seen.

"I never thought I would be so hungry for a piece of bread," Ethel Owens, a nurse from Maine, told Betty Belanger. Betty, the New Hampshire nurse, had joined the army because of an "enlist-together-and-stay-together" promise that quickly went bad when the friend she'd enlisted with, Irene Labrie, got sent to Hawaii and Betty to France.

Down the way, Dottie tied a bandage around a can of C-rations and lowered it into a boiling pot of water. Above, anti-aircraft fire flashed, the sky ablaze with "ack-ack." For every pinkish tracer bullet a nurse could see, four more were zinging through the air that she couldn't.

"I'm going to go scare up some coffee," said Monty Montague. She was joined by Carolea "Tex" Roe, the lone nurse from west of the Mississippi—lanky, blond, and, at the moment, petrified.

A few minutes later, the nurses heard it: the buzz of planes far louder than what they'd been hearing. Monty and Tex were on their way back to join the other off-duty nurses, having just filled their canteens with a new kind of instant coffee called "Nescafé."

"Hit the dirt!" someone yelled. Nurses skittered into foxholes; weary minds jolted into panic modes. Bullets peppered the ground, then stopped. Another burst tattered the makeshift camp. The sound of the planes diminished. Betty resumed breathing.

"Aren't we the damned fools," muttered Tex, her back to Monty in a foxhole. Monty was too stunned to answer. All she knew was that they'd been in Normandy only one full day and nearly been killed. And Carolea was already talking about wanting to go back home to Texas.

In a nearby foxhole lay a lone nurse. It was Frances Slanger. She was still. She was splattered in red. She was asleep in the Normandy night, baptized by war and the blood of the soldiers fighting it. Above, artillery guns pounded and planes whined, making the sound of Boston's trolleys and trains seem almost appealing by comparison.

As the streetcar rolled away from her, south down Harrison Avenue, Frances stood in front of Boston City Hospital. She was on a mission both exciting and frightening. Exciting because she was venturing beyond where she had been. Frightening because she did so against her parents' wishes, as if even stepping into this building would somehow taint her as a traitor. And because it cut against the grain of her education as well.

The High School of Practical Arts, an all-girls school on the corner of Greenville and Winthrop Streets, stood about a mile and a half south of where Frances lived, near the Dudley Street Elevated Station. Its teachers, when they could be heard over the groaning and grinding of train cars on the Dudley turn-around, liked to remind students that the school aspired to strike a new note in secondary education. "It is conducted," noted a 1925 brochure on the school, "in the belief that woman's highest calling is that of a homemaker."

Frances, at age seventeen, began at the school in the fall of 1930. She studied hard. She took weekend hikes, sometimes to the top of nearby Mount McKay, with a handful of classmates who called themselves the Aderoosk Club. She helped deliver fruit. And she buried her nose in books and magazines.

She had, her poetry attested, the highest regard for her mother and the woman's role as a homemaker. She understood the link between work and love and how she'd been the beneficiary of such love from her mother: "As long as she is well and strong/And works and sings the whole day long . . . You do not have a care!" She'd even been happy to see Sally, now twenty-three, marry James Sidman the previous Christmas Day. But if Practical Arts strived to make women homemakers, Frances found herself drawn to a different calling. She stood in front of the Boston City Hospital School of Nursing and imagined herself as part of that calling. She walked inside and timidly requested an audience with Miss Daily, a nursing supervisor.

Did she have an appointment? No, she did not. But soon she was sitting in the office of Miss Daily, asking what she must do to become a nurse. What could she do to increase her chances of gaining admission to the School of Nursing? Could she do some volunteer work in the meantime? Come back, Miss Daily told her, when you've graduated from high school.

Later, Frances took a greater adventure, as far from the South End as she probably had ever gone on her own, to the convalescent home of the Children's Hospital in Wellesley Hills, twenty miles northwest of Boston. "I always have been fond of children and I thought I'd like to specialize along that line of work," she had written in a letter of introduction. But when she visited the home, a nursing supervisor said: Come back when you've graduated from high school. Frances got back on a streetcar and headed for home. Slouched down in a seat, she watched the world pass by outside.

In the spring of 1931, a Practical Arts English teacher named Miss Shaw was preparing to read to students as she did each Friday afternoon when she realized the desk was vacant—again. It was Frances Slanger's. And she knew exactly where the girl was: working a fruit route with her father. It was hardly a proper substitute for Emerson or Shakespeare, but the Depression, Miss Shaw realized, was changing people's priorities.

Wall Street's crash in October 1929 had plunged the country into economic catastrophe. In Boston, people stood in breadlines. Peddlers with three months' growth went to sleep beneath their carts on cold nights and never woke up. Idle workers waited for boats at the fish pier to get unsalable scraps of codfish. Mr.

Schiff, a butcher in nearby Dorchester, learned to slice an eighth of a pound of corned beef into six paper-thin pieces so everyone in a family could have one.

For David Slanger, making money on a fruit route became like finding berries in a picked-over field. Who had money for luxuries like oranges and grapes when some people were scrounging spilled coal from the sides of the Boston & Albany rails to keep the house warm? But selling fruit was all Frances's father knew and having Frances along with him helped the route go faster. The more distance he could cover, the better chance he had of at least coming back with *something*.

As the Depression hardened, some Practical Arts students quit school altogether, their parents finding it difficult to justify education when a child could be, say, collecting *Boston Globe*s left on the streetcars so the newspapers could be resold. Frances tried to do both: work and attend school. In three years of high school, she missed eighty-seven days, largely because she was still helping her father on the fruit route as an eighteen-year-old.

"Good morning, *Faigie*," Milton Zola said one morning from atop his father's fruit cart, smoke from the fires of the homeless shrouding the streets. Milton wondered if his "big sister" would grow old and gray as the fruit peddler's daughter.

"Morning, *Motle*," said Frances, hardly looking up.

Because of the fruit route, Frances was forever playing catch-up, memorizing spelling words while making fruit deliveries or catching a few winks of sleep in the school library. She continued to write. She continued to contribute to the school's literary magazine, *The Shuttle*. She continued to inspire herself with her own words: "When in school, should you miss a test/Make it up and your conscience will rest."

Frances's passion for writing was more impressive than her execution. "You write *'con amore'* " (Italian for "with love") wrote a teacher on one of her papers. "There is in the physical structure of the story, however, certain oddities of construction and vocabulary, which unfortunately mar the ultimate effect." The teacher recommended Frances read no less than six books, including the entire Old Testament "over and over." Frances could only shake her head. If her early years in America infused her with the idea of possibilities, her high school years ushered in a harsher reality. It was one thing to be told to read William Shepherd's *Manual and Model for English Composition*. It was quite another, amid 4 A.M. wakeups and finger-numbing cold, to actually *do* it.

As the Depression worsened, her father demanded more time from her on the route; nineteen absences as a sophomore turned into thirty-six as a junior. As a senior, she was having to cram five days of lessons into three or four days at school. In the fall of her senior year, she also missed some school to have surgery for a deviated septum, correcting a crooked nose. In some classes, Bs and As became Cs. At school, classmates disappeared like soldiers in battle, quitting to help rustle food or because the family was moving in with family members elsewhere.

Come back when you've graduated from high school. A diploma was beginning to look like a mountain too high, but it was a mountain she had to climb in order to have a chance at getting into nursing school. She heard the whistles of the few factories still in operation. Perhaps they called for her. Perhaps in this time and place, even the tiniest dream was too large to come true. Perhaps her destiny was packing olives at F. P. Adams & Company on Dover Street or stuffing envelopes at Emerson Piano Company on Harrison.

At night, up on the roof, Frances looked at the star-studded sky and rhythmically petted Yip-Yip, wondering where in the world she belonged. And who was she, really? The past seemed to whisper that she was the fruit peddler's daughter, the nonstop "go-between," someone who rushes here and there, running errands for her Yiddish-speaking parents, but never really fitting at either point, so destined to live her life as the flat, ordinary line in between.

She despised that idea: *ordinary*. But everywhere she turned, that was the message: Her life was as predestined as a windup toy. She tried to believe it wasn't true; she sensed she could be *more*. The poets and writers told her as much. "Do not be afraid to be different," she had read in a piece by Bill MacKellar. "Every person varies in character, just as each one has a different face and body. Be content, then, to make something out of the character that Nature gives you."

But how can you make something out of that character if others won't let you *be* anything but what they say you are? As she looked up at the sky, Frances Slanger realized she wasn't up on that roof after all. She was still back on Ellis Island. She was, like her parakeet, a prisoner of sorts. More than a decade had passed since she had come to America and yet, in some ways, she was still that little girl in the cage, being detained by the authorities.

In Oradour-sur-Glane, 250 miles southeast of where the Forty-fifth had dug in, a farmer named Hyvernaud went in search of his two sons—Marchel, twelve, and André, six—who attended the boys school in the village but hadn't returned home Saturday night. It was daybreak on Sunday morning, June 11, 1944.

First, he smelled the smoke, then—*"Oh, my God!"*—he saw Oradour-sur-Glane: burned to the ground. What could this be? He ran to the village. He found only one son, André, in the church. The boy was half charred. One of his legs was completely out of joint and twisted back. His throat was cut through. The father bent over and kissed his dead son on the cheek. The man could not find his other son so he went back home and told his wife. They brought back some sheets. They wrapped up André's body and carried him home.

From outlying areas, word spread. Others started making their way to Oradour-sur-Glane. A group of women who lived outside the village and whose children had gone to school the previous day searched for them in the woods, thinking they'd perhaps gotten lost coming home. But a man and woman—a couple named Leveques—stumbled toward them, from the direction of the village. The woman wailed; the man tore at his shirt, ripping it apart piece by piece.

"Don't hunt any longer," he said, his face in anguish. "They've all been burned. I've seen it—I've seen it. They've burned our children in the church."

Across the village, fires smoldered amid charred concrete, brick walls, and the few cars villagers owned. Fifteenth-century structures lay in ruins. Business signs, for the most part, remained unscathed: the Hotel Milord, the Café du Chene, and others labeled simply "Baker's" and "Hairdresser." Dogs and cats and farm animals wandered aimlessly through the rubble. One corpse, that of a man, was stuck to a fence, the Germans having jokingly tethered a horse to his hand. The remains of a mother, father, and child were found stuffed inside a baker's oven.

The church's roof was gone. Inside, broken statues lay on the ground. The acrid smell of burnt flesh choked the throats of those who had come to identify bodies. Two children lay in the confessional, holding each other around the neck, in death. Several babies' remains were found still cradled in their mothers' arms. Nearby, a young child had been crammed in the priest's privy, its skull crushed. On the wall: a bloodstain. All of it done while the nurses of the Forty-fifth came ashore—and done by German soldiers who would soon join the Battle of Normandy themselves.

Only fifty-two of the 642 bodies were identifiable; the rest were either too charred to recognize or simply couldn't be found. On the side of the church hung an iron-sculpted crucifix, Christ's head bowed in anguish. As the few remaining townspeople fanned out throughout the village, they found a blood-stained letter from a woman, dated the day of the tragedy, that included the line, "I feel fine now. For me the sun shines here now."

While people searched through the rubble on this Sunday morning, a group of German soldiers entered the village and furiously began digging shallow graves here and there, trying to hide the evidence. They piled bodies in basements and covered them with debris. But after a few hours, they realized it was a futile attempt and left. A dead man's hand was left sticking out of the ground, another gruesome validation of an evil Frances Slanger had known was at work in the world but, in Normandy, was now seeing for herself in the eyes of dead soldiers.

"There is no priest, minister, or rabbi to comfort the wounded and administer last rites to the dying," she'd written in the early part of the war. But now, as the Normandy dawn revealed the carnage of battle that darkness hides, nurses, Frances among them, were emerging as those comforters. Before the war was over, the same GIs who'd catcalled such women as they came ashore would see them differently. They'd begin calling them Nightingales. American Nightingales.

CHAPTER 5

*It is not the critic who counts; not the man who points out
how the strong man stumbled or where the doer of deeds
could have done better. The credit belongs to the man who is
actually in the arena; whose face is marred by dust and sweat
and blood.*

—ANONYMOUS,
FOUND IN FRANCES SLANGER'S CHAPBOOK

Capt. Joseph P. Shoham, the Second Platoon's dentist, mess
hall czar, and self-appointed naturalist, was on a food forage
in a Normandy farmyard when he saw them. He was looking for
fresh eggs, already considered a rare and coveted delicacy in these
early days of war. Then came the delightful distraction: three
dead stag beetles. He found them next to the maggot-ridden body
of a German soldier that was slouched against a barn and deep in
decay. The beetles were on the ground, not far from the soldier's
steel belt buckle and its *Gott mit uns* ("God with us") inscription.

Shoham pressed a handkerchief over his nose to mask
death's stench and bent down on one knee. He grimaced slightly—he had a bad back—and reached toward the ground next to
the dead soldier. Carefully, he flicked the dead beetles into a
cigar box. After a quick search of the shell-pocked farmyard

turned up no eggs, he headed back to the Second Platoon's camp a few hundred feet away, where doctors and nurses had been reunited after their separate landings five days before. Shoham proudly showed off his find.

"Them for dinner or breakfast?" cracked a private lying on his back, head propped on his helmet.

"Don't matter," chimed in a second, between bites of a Normandy apple. "Be better'n anything else we've had."

As head of the mess tent, Shoham wanted to bloody both wise guys' mouths but, as a dentist, had far too much regard for his own teeth, which would be imperiled were he to start throwing punches; Jack Dempsey he was not. Instead, he cleared his throat.

"The Captain Joseph P. Shoham World War II Beetles Collection," he announced, "has begun."

Frances, sitting on an overturned wash tin while brushing her hair, stopped briefly to offer staccato applause. Shoham smiled and bowed to her in appreciation. "You won't find these kind back home," he said.

For Shoham, "back home" was the Bronx, ironic for a man enthralled with nature. But, then, Shoham had a certain quirkiness about him, from eloping with his wife, Ethel, and not telling anybody for fifteen months that they were married to running the mess hall with General MacArthur bravado.

Twenty-nine years old, a year younger than Frances, he was slight of build, round-jawed, large-eared—a Jew who hated Germans as much as he loved butterflies, beetles, and just about anything else he could collect and categorize. He had enlisted while in his senior year of college at Columbia University Dental School in New York and thought he'd be spending his army days pulling teeth and filling cavities. Instead, with dental work in light demand, he was asked to draw straws for Second Platoon mess boss. He lost.

"Welcome to the army, Yank," said one of the winners, among many enlisted men from the South who would become Shoham's mess crew—and be referred to by him as "Rebels" or just plain "Rebs."

Shoham, more than most, was an observer, not only a student of bugs and butterflies, but of people as well. In his mind, he had already classified most of the Second Platoon: Maj. Herman Lord, of Detroit, Michigan, the frumpy but friendly doctor in charge of the seventy-five person platoon; Capt. Fred "Mike" Michalove, the softhearted southerner who was the platoon's administrator; doctors John Bonzer, Herman Hirsh, and Isadore Schwartz; nurses Frances Slanger, Christine Cox, Elizabeth Powers, and Margaret Bowler; and, of course, the five dozen enlisted men, including his circle of Rebs.

Shoham had already observed that the enlisted men were suspicious of the nurses and a tad jealous that the women were officers and they weren't. That his tent mate, Bonzer—Shoham called him *Hunzeczech*, meaning "Little John," to kid him about his small size and his Czechoslovakian descent—had fallen hard for that nurse from Wisconsin in the First Platoon, Sallylou. That even though he was better known as "a big teddy bear," there wasn't a finer doctor in the Forty-fifth than Isadore "Tiny" Schwartz. And that there was something curiously inviting about this nurse Frances Slanger, though he wasn't quite sure what. All he knew was that, among the Forty-fifth, there was nobody else like her. Jewish doctors were plentiful—Bonzer was the only non-Jew among the Second Platoon's doctors—but a Jewish nurse? In war or out of war, they were as rare as ajax butterflies in the Bronx. Shoham wondered just who she was and what she was doing here.

It was June 15, 1944, the first day the platoon had been able to take a breather since hitting the beach five days earlier. After the Forty-fifth Field Hospital's three platoons had gone their separate ways, the Second was bivouacked near a stone farm-house at Audoville la Hubert, about two miles from the first lib-erated village in France, Ste.-Mère-Église. Low clouds shrouded the fields and trees of France. What was emerging as one of the wettest Normandy Junes in recent memory had given the Allies a short reprieve, at least for the moment.

A handful of enlisted men, hands blistered from digging slit trenches, slept or shared bottles of Calvados, an apple brandy they'd found and happily dubbed "white lightning." Those trying to sleep tried to ignore the distant chatter of machine-gun fire, the buzz of bees, and the odd sound of laughter. It erupted in a supply tent after a private with wire cutters snapped the bands on a tightly packed pallet of sanitary napkins for the nurses—and they sprang into the air as if launched from a jack-in-the-box.

While most of the six dozen people in the Second Platoon relaxed, day-shift doctors and nurses inside the medical tents continued the incessant quest to fix broken soldiers. Smoke rose from the skeletal remains of the villages beyond. And a handful of French children in scuffed wooden shoes watched enlisted men outside the surgical tent stuff the bloody uniforms of the dead and wounded, along with soiled sheets, into canvas bags. At night, enlisted men would go through the uniforms to remove any stray ammunition, then, for sanitary reasons, burn the clothes.

THE FORTY-FIFTH's three platoons had been bouncing around the Normandy coast like pinballs. After the Allied success on D-Day, there had been talk of celebrating Fourth of July in Paris, 145 miles to the east. But most fighting units were bogged down in the Normandy hedgerows, not far from the beaches they'd won on June 6.

The hedgerows were proving hugely advantageous to the

Germans. These mounds of earth, which had been used for defense since the days of the Romans, rose up to six feet high and were used to separate farmers' fields from one another. Fortified by deep-rooted bushes or trees, they stalled American tanks and hid German troops, guns, and tanks equally well. The Forty-fifth got its daily customers from the result of skirmishes between German and American soldiers playing deadly games of hide and seek in honeycombs of hedgerows. U.S. troops measured their advance by fields, not miles.

The ultimate goal was to break out of Normandy and push the Germans east to their homeland. A few miles behind the front lines, some eighty-eight field hospitals, such as the Forty-fifth, would follow the surge. First, though, the Americans needed to push north, up the Contentin Peninsula that stretched, thumblike, into the English Channel, and wrest the major deep-water port of Cherbourg from the Germans. But in a low range of hills running parallel to the beach, the Germans dug in deep; they knew that if they allowed a "breakout" the Americans would find no resistance between Normandy and the German border.

Shoham unfastened a trunk, looking for kitchen supplies he'd been unable to find. "Hear about our trip across the Channel?" he said to Frances. "Came over on a British pleasure ship. Got served K-rations by porters in *tuxedos*. Those Brits know how to host a war, huh?"

Frances, no student of small talk, particularly with men, hesitated for a moment. "No, I *hadn't* heard that—but I did hear about Isadore," she said. "The same thing happened to me coming ashore."

"He just disappeared," said Shoham. "Stepped in a shell hole and, poof, gone. Swallowed by the sea. Hard to lose a guy that tall. We were lucky to save him."

She thought about Isadore Schwartz, the way he towered over her but never talked down to her. "Glad you did."

Frances had met Shoham and Schwartz in England, where the Forty-fifth had been billeted in Upton-on-Severn, 144 miles northwest of London. There, an elderly woman who ran a pub learned that Shoham liked sweet wine; she got a bottle from the local priest and Shoham invited Frances, Schwartz, and a few others to join him. On Friday evenings in Upton, Schwartz had led Sabbath services for the Jews in the outfit—Frances, Shoham, Michalove, Hirsh, and a handful of others. Shoham thought it interesting that Tiny and Frances were becoming such close friends; Schwartz was six-foot-three, Slanger only a shade over five feet.

Now, in Audoville la Hubert, Shoham closed the trunk; his utensils must be elsewhere. "So, Slanger," he said, "how'd you wind up as a nurse?"

THE STREETCAR rattled south of Boston, then east. Frances, slouched low in the seat, watched block after block of boarded-up brick buildings, homeless men asleep on park benches, and wooden shanties, the refuse of a Depression showing no signs of ending. She had managed to graduate from the High School of Practical Arts on June 23, 1933. Three days later, here she was, heart pounding with anticipation, though not the kind of anticipation she'd hoped for. After fifteen minutes, the Irish driver drew the car to a halt at her stop.

"Bickford Street!" he yelled.

Frances stepped outside and saw it: the factory. She had gotten work in the stockroom of Massachusetts Knitting Mills. Her job was to pack hosiery into boxes and stamp them. She was to make $13 a week.

With Frances now only weeks away from her twentieth birthday, her parents would have her follow Sally's lead, find a man, and settle down. But if she had thought herself too old to keep working the fruit route with her father, this was a satisfactory alternative—at least in her parents' eyes. By now, her father's health and the family's financial plight were growing worse. Beyond a nagging cough, David had been diagnosed with prostate gland hypertrophy, a urinary disease that would likely curb his ability to do the entire fruit route each day. He was forever having to go to the bathroom. Frances's money from the factory became the family's financial salvation.

Amid summer's deepening heat, she took the streetcar home each night to the family flat on Oneida Street, and wrote and read. She was a lucky girl to have such a job in these hard times, her parents would remind her. Frances found it hard to feel lucky about packing socks into a box. But this is what is expected of you, her father would say. As Morris Zola had always said, this is your *freedom*—"even if you are digging ditches."

Except Frances dreamed of a deeper freedom. She wanted something more—and not the "more" sought by the other Jewish girls: the clothes, the house, the *yichus*—the inherent nobility or distinction associated with marrying a Jewish man of means. And not the "more" of Jewish men: the job, the prestige, the great sums of money that would buy them fine houses in Roxbury or Dorchester and status in the eyes of their colleagues. Frances wanted to matter in a different way, a way that veered from the course that the cultural currents had set for her. She wanted to help those who couldn't help themselves, like little Sammie Yanoff, the family friend down the street, who'd just died of polio at age twelve.

Since her childhood in Poland, Frances had gone where she was told to go, whether by soldiers, immigration officials, teachers, or parents. Now, at age twenty, she followed the crowd onto the streetcar and to the factory each morning. She worked. She came home.

Do not be afraid to be different. Bill MacKellar's inspirational words were carefully clipped and pasted in her chapbook, like a star that burned brighter than the rest, somehow meant only for her. Still, she got up and went to work at the factory. She worked. She came home. She read.

Think for yourself and go where that thinking may lead, even though it be in the opposite direction of the crowd. Do not be one of the herd. . . .

She got up and went to work at the factory. She worked. She came home. She read.

Avoid being eccentric or peculiar, but if your conscience supports your course, lay that course into uncharted seas without fear. Remember that every great movement, every reformation, began with a minority. It is the minority in every age that makes history. . . .

She got up and went to work at the factory. She worked. She came home. Then one day she did something that would change her life forever. It was a Wednesday, June 30, a sweltering day on which Boston's temperature reached 99 degrees. The skies, pent up with summer heat, darkened. Thunderclouds billowed. By evening, lightning flashed over the city. Amid the summer storm, Frances did it: She filled out an application for the Boston City Hospital School of Nursing, then mailed it the next day. Later, she wrote to Della Currier, superintendent of the School of Nursing.

Dear Miss Currier,

I have mailed my application to you and now I am not quite certain whether I am doing right writing this letter.

If I am not, please forgive me.

At present, I weigh one hundred and eight pounds and I'm five feet one inches tall. My health is considered good.

I came to America thirteen years ago and am now a true American citizen. Miss Currier, it isn't a very simple task in trying to tell you why I wish to be a nurse, although I have many reasons for wishing so.

This isn't just a sudden thought on my part. I have thought it for many, many years. I have always loved to comfort those who were sick. I realize fully that I must give my time up to work and study and I am prepared to go into it heart and soul.

I am looking into the future. Some people say one should not look ahead but I must. After all, I am the future and although things do not come out the way I try to plan them—look ahead and plan I must. Even when I was a very little girl I used to say I was going to be a nurse. My people used to laugh at me, but now they are willing that I should be a nurse. To put my real reason into a few words: I want to serve they who are less fortunate than I.

Thank you very much for reading so patiently and may I hope to hear from you.

Sincerely,
Frances Slanger

How willing "her people" were to let her be a nurse was debatable. Asked on a reference-check form if the applicant had any faults, Practical Arts teacher Marguerite C. Cronan wrote: "I know of no outstanding faults, unless it is in her persistence to get a higher education in spite of the opposition of her parents."

Frances so desperately wanted to be a nurse that she wasn't as forthcoming as she might have been on such matters. On her own registration application, she was asked, "Are your eyesight and hearing perfect?" Despite having worn thick glasses for years, Frances wrote "yes." But if she would allow nothing to deter her diminutive dreams, others wouldn't be as intent on helping her reach them. After giving Frances a physical examination on August 31, 1933, Dr. Joel Ginsburg was, in an evaluation, asked to assess Frances's "general appearance as to capabilities of making a nurse."

"Fair," he wrote.

At Boston City Hospital, about a mile southwest of the Slanger flat, Della Currier perused Frances's application and letters of recommendation. One Practical Arts teacher, Irene Watson, had described Frances as a "very courteous and conscientious student . . . highly intelligent and sensible . . . bright-minded . . . ambitious . . . honorable. . . ."

Cronan wrote that Frances was "one of my very best pupils and a rock of sense. With her earnestness of purpose and her general ability she ought to be a success. She has been most anxious for a higher education and had difficulty achieving it . . . I highly recommend her and I hope you will give her a chance. . . ."

That's all Frances wanted—a chance. And so, as she worked at the knitting mills in the summer of 1933, she waited for one. A handful of concerns hindered her hopes, among them having attended a high school that was training young women to be homemakers and nothing else. She hadn't had a single math, general science, or biology class, and had gotten mainly Cs in the one year of chemistry she'd taken.

Meanwhile, she may well have wondered if her Jewishness would be used against her, particularly if a number of other Jewish girls applied—not likely, given the cultural taboo, but still possible. Boston City Hospital's School of Nursing may not have had written policies regarding Jewish and black candidates, but anti-Semitism and racism lurked in Boston's shadows. Quota systems existed for Jewish medical students in many city hospitals and Boston City's nursing school allowed only two "colored girls" per term.

Frances's application was accepted. She was to report for the winter session in February 1934, a possibility that, for a young woman not used to approval, seemed straight from a fairy tale. But her parents did not share her excitement. Where was Frances going to get the $21 necessary for textbooks and $35 for a uniform? Student nurses lived in a dormitory and paid no tuition; instead, they were given a $10-a-month stipend in exchange for serving as nurses-in-training their first year. Still, they didn't get that until their third month. Meanwhile, Frances was giving up the factory's $13-a-week that was the family's main income.

Frances wrote back to Miss Currier, thanking her for the opportunity but expressing concern at the required fees. "Is there any way that I might lessen the expense?" she wrote. "If there were just a little bit it would be deeply appreciated. However, if not, I shall try to manage."

The nursing supervisor wrote back and said, in essence: *try to manage.* Frances decided she would. She would scrape up child care work from some woman still fortunate enough to have a job. She would make it work. She would forge herself a future.

TATTERED SUITCASE in hand, Frances stood at the corner of Harrison Avenue and East Springfield Street, facing the five-story Vose House, the brick student nurses' dormitory across the street from the hospital. She stared at the round-arched entryway She was *here.*

Inside, she found her room was far nicer, and far more private, than anything she'd ever lived in. Like the rooms of her forty-seven classmates, it had a single bed, a throw rug, a dresser, a cast-iron radiator, and two wicker rocking chairs. Down the hall was a swimming pool. For Frances, Vose House might as well have been the queen's palace. Across the street stood the stately seventy-eight-year-old Boston City Hospital, its domed administration building flanked by French-inspired wings fluted with elegant mansard roofs.

Frances, lying on her bed, began reading the school's

guidelines, which quickly rubbed the glow off her arrival. The first part posed no threat: Student nurses had to be willing to postpone marriage and motherhood. Frances, hardly pinup material, didn't have suitors lined up from here to Dorchester Bay. The second part caused her pause, however: "Nurses, when called, must report promptly and bring with them means of returning to their homes should they not successfully complete their probationary term."

Once again, she had to prove herself worthy, the phrase "probationary term" hovering above her like a vulture. And she had to do so in a military-like atmosphere. Nursing school at Boston City Hospital, Frances soon found, was a caste system whose founding testament, if unwritten, was as black and white as the *Boston Globe*. Supervisors were God. Students weren't.

Frances saw some nursing supervisors as virtual drill sergeants in dresses, letter-of-the-law school marms who saw the crumbling of Western civilization in every rules infraction. Two nurses had been suspended for listening to a radio. One student nurse had been caught smoking in the lavatory and a supervisor recommended her dismissal—"not because of the smoking . . . but because this is the first time that we know of an occurrence of this kind, and it would seem advisable to make an example of the case to prevent any repetition of same. . . ." The nursing staff was known to search students' suitcases or drawers for articles it believed may have been stolen, until informed by the City of Boston's law department that, without a warrant, that was illegal.

One instructor in particular cracked down on student nurses with particular fervor and subtle glee. Her name was Anna Holland. So feared was the woman that when a classmate of Frances's, Hazelle Ferguson, heard the phone ring while Nurse Holland was on night duty, she considered it a call from the devil himself. Nurse Holland, who was in her fifties, thrived on her position of authority and preyed on those who didn't bow low enough to that authority. None may have bowed with less enthusiasm than Frances Slanger.

Whether aimed at Frances's attitude, educational naïveté, or Jewishness, Holland fired consistent criticism at her. Holland thought Frances was a lone wolf who had no business becoming a nurse. "Miss Slanger works well under supervision but is not capable," wrote Holland on November 17, 1934. She reported that Frances was "blundering, slow, irresponsible and resented criticism." Later, she marked Frances down for being nervous, immature, self-centered, insincere and "questioning authority."

In writing, Frances vented freely about her distaste for power-hungry supervisors such as Holland. "She towers above you majestically and starts to criticize everything in no uncertain terms from the beginning of her tour until, with a snort of disgust, she marches off the ward," she wrote of her "nightmare supervisor," whom she affectionately labeled a "snoopervisor."

> Give me the supervisor who will quietly call you aside to reprimand you for something and does not show her superiority by scolding or belittling you in front of an audience of student nurses, doctors, or outside visitors— not to mention patients. Above all, give me the supervisor who will occasionally say how nice the ward looks as she smiles. . . . Please do not let me come in contact with the type who, when under the impression that you have done a wrong, quickly runs to the telephone to report it to the matron's office before giving you a chance to explain.

As much as Frances may have despised the woman, Holland had a huge say in whether she would graduate. The frostiness between the two grew even colder. Beyond Holland, Frances struggled with the glut of information she was having to know.

Frances had jumped into a program that her high school education had done little to prepare her for—and soon found herself
struggling to stay afloat in a sea of anatomy, physiology, chemistry, pharmaceuticals, personal hygiene, and nutrition.

She was in class or on duty sixty to seventy hours a week,
supervisors giving time off with only great reluctance. She was
taking written and oral exams. And she was thrown into on-the-
job training, which taught her in a hurry that nursing was far
more than taking temperatures and fluffing pillows. One night a
male patient at Boston City went berserk and began swinging
wildly at nurses who tried to restrain him. "I had my shirt torn
and there are marks of his teeth on my side where the patient bit
me," reported the orderly. Another orderly was fired after being
caught one night on a fire escape, peeping in rooms. "It seems to
me that he is not a desirable person to have in the hospital at
night," wrote a nursing supervisor.

Frances's test scores were meager, her body weary, her
mind jangled. She was overloaded with the dos and don'ts of
medicine and the more onerous ticky-tack rules of nursing
supervisors who spit them out like machine-gun bullets. Among
them: "Riding or coasting on the transfer truss is absolutely prohibited. Any infraction of this will result in dismissal." And: "In
the event that a patient to whom whiskey has been dispensed
dies or is discharged, it shall be the duty of the nurse in charge
of the ward to send back to the Dispensary any whiskey that may
be left over."

By spring 1934, Frances's stomach was knotted in worry, her
"happy-to-be-here" smile all but gone. It wasn't that she feared
getting beat out for the $5 prize awarded annually to the
highest-ranking pupil in operating room technique; that was a
given. It was that she feared not making it past her probationary

term, period. On evaluations from teachers, she scored extremely high in four areas: "sympathy toward patients," "dignity,"
"courteousness," and "accepting criticism." But she struggled in
terms of "speed," "adaptability," "reliability," and "sense of
humor."

"She is still a little 'in the fog' about the routine of so large
an undertaking," wrote one instructor.

Frances slipped past the probationary scare, but began
struggling in other ways. At times, she clashed with fellow students who didn't treat patients as seriously or as compassionately
as she thought they should. At times, she clashed with supervisors over priorities. Frances believed some supervisors were
more concerned about wrinkle-free beds than the patients *in*
those beds—and expressed as much on occasion. "You mean
well," a Nurse Cotter told her, "but you spend more time doing
small tasks that do not concern you and letting some important
things go."

Midway through the three-year program, Frances was convinced that broken people could not be put back together again
as if they were assembly-line parts. They needed to be nurtured,
given hope, comforted—regardless of who they were, how much
money they had, or what color they were. On the hospital's
rooftop, where nurses often went for a breath of fresh air or to
rock babies, Frances sometimes coddled a black infant, which
merited a few looks of disgust in a hospital where race was
clearly an issue. Of the forty-eight nurses in Slanger's Class of
1937, only one, Hazelle Ferguson, was black. Nursing supervisors were forever writing memos to supervisors, fretting that
they'd received yet more applications from "colored girls" who
kept asking, as one letter said, "why their applications are not being acted upon."

"I am submitting to you the application of Miss Imogene
Roundtree," wrote one nursing supervisor. "She is a young

woman who made application in person, and although her complexion was fairer than most negro people, she showed evidence of belonging to that race. You will note that the principal of the high school says she is a member of the negro race. I am asking you for advice."

Frances had a heart for those whom the world did not, dating back to her days in Lødz when a Jew might be spit on by a German soldier—or Polish citizen—for simply being a Jew. She had taken care of her wheelchair-bound neighbor boy, Samuel Yanoff, when others her age were lounging in Franklin Park. At nursing school, she took the case studies that other nurses would pass on, including five-year-old Thelma Toye, whose mother was white and her father Mongolian.

What Frances loved best about all this was simply seeing people get better; she had always been a sucker for a happy ending. In one of her short stories, she wrote of a "Mr. Chauncy," a well-to-do, if miserable, man. He begins Christmas Eve as a Scrooge-like character who, hearing the sound of carol-singing children, tells his wife he's glad the two of them have not started a family. By the end of the evening, he has fallen in love with, and adopted, a "roguish little boy" who has been mysteriously left in a basket on the Chauncys' snow-swept porch.

It was the same way in the hospital: She believed miracles like that could happen, and that she could be part of them—but not if heartless supervisors kept lording their power over her. What mattered to Frances, simply, was justice. Fairness. People. She could slough off a C+ on a chemistry exam. She could rationalize a so-so dry-mop job on a ward floor. What she couldn't accept was people failing one another. Nor could she accept a world that was growing increasingly cold.

By now, Frances had seen the newsreels of the Hitler Youth, their arms outstretched in salute to the Führer. She had heard of the pro-Nazi rallies in New York. Now this: a German zeppelin floating over Roxbury one summer night, stirring a sense of fascination and fear from the people below. It was named the *Graf Zeppelin* and had four swastikas emblazoned on its tail, each the size of a roadside billboard.

The airships had been regular guests over America since 1929. Americans, in fact, seemed more enamored of them than German citizens. Jews, however, weren't as taken by the sensation in the sky. In Roxbury's Franklin Park, a group of young Jews gathered in a circle and danced the hora in defiance as the ship floated above. Others, Frances perhaps among them, felt a slight chill as the zeppelin eased through the darkness, its belly light sweeping the ground below.

Eva Slanger heard footsteps pounding up the stairs to the Oneida Street flat. In burst Frances, who threw herself on the couch in tears. When calmed down by her mother, she sobbed forth the story: how she'd been reprimanded by a supervisor. More than reprimanded, *ridiculed*. For what? For spending too much time with sick children on her ward.

How could she be criticized for caring too much? Isn't that why she had become a nurse in the first place? Isn't that the whole idea of this profession?

Perhaps she wasn't meant to be a nurse. Perhaps she belonged back in the factory line, where supervisors wouldn't have to worry about her getting too "attached" to her work. Perhaps she should march into Miss Holland's office the next day and tell her what some had been telling her for years: that nursing wasn't for her.

Instead, perhaps buoyed by her own poetry—"Life is much too short, yes much / Stop your brooding tears and such . . ."—she returned to Boston City and continued her pursuit of becoming a nurse, even if she seriously doubted whether that day would ever come. Some of the twenty-nine instructors either found Frances lacking or simply didn't like her—and channeled that dislike into their evaluations. Some didn't believe her qualified to be a nurse—and did more to dissuade her than to encourage her.

"Miss Slanger antagonized a great many people," wrote Holland. "Miss Slanger is very aggressive," wrote Anne Crowley. "She antagonized people because she does not know her place."

The bulk of criticism came from two nurses—Holland and Crowley—who rarely had anything good to say about anybody. Hazelle Ferguson found Holland "a horror." Crowley was cut from the same cloth. Once, Crowley so thoroughly chastised Hazelle that the student nurse—who was tough enough to be among the first "colored" nurses to break the school's two-a-year quota—fled to the bathroom in tears.

In the end, Rose Foster, acting superintendent of nurses, had the final say in whether Frances Slanger would graduate. In February 1937, with Frances's three years now up, it was time for a decision. Foster reviewed the reports of supervisors such as Holland and Crowley, then others, including this from Helen Sullivan: "Slanger does very good work. She is very conscientious and very sympathetic with her patients. She shows a marked interest in her work."

"She always follows instructions," wrote Alice Senior. "She is liked by her patients."

"She is reliable and neat and is a rapid worker," wrote O. Ferguson. "Her manner is professional at all times. She has initiative and good executive ability and shows intelligence and culture."

Foster's final evaluation of the young student blew like a blustery wind, here and there. Frances was inclined to do things her own way, Foster wrote. She was "very aggressive and did not always use good judgment or tact." And "she had some executive ability but no leadership or teaching ability. . . ."

But Foster's final word was this: Frances Slanger was worthy of being a nurse. On February 23, 1937, Frances graduated from Boston City Hospital's School of Nursing. Whether her father embraced the idea of her being a nurse, her mother's reticence melted. On the roof of the hospital, Eva feigned illness for a comical photo, her daughter "worriedly" checking the "patient's" pulse—not the kind of thing a disapproving mother might do.

Soon thereafter, Frances passed the state exams. The confirmation arrived at the Slangers' flat in a letter with a two-cent stamp: Once "Freidel Schlanger," then "Frances Slanger," she was now "Frances Slanger, R.N." She had heeded the advice from MacKellar, the writer, to sail the uncharted seas.

IN MARCH 1938, Austria buckled to Nazi Germany in the blink of an eye. Jewish men and women, rifles at their backs, were forced to get down on their knees and scrub graffiti off the sidewalks. German soldiers laughed. This was their country now and the Jews were their slaves.

The same month, Frances, now a full-time nurse, cut out an article from the *Boston Sunday Advertiser* that had been written by Rabbi Joseph Shubow of Boston. In it, he decried the evil of Hitler and bemoaned America's collective yawn in response. "A sacred task confronts the keepers of civilization and religion," he wrote. "Let us unite to curb, muzzle and silence the Madman of Europe before his ravings turn the whole world into an insane asylum." Few listened, but among those who did was Frances.

Eight months later, in Germany, Hitler's forces unleashed their anti-Jewish wrath in what would be known as "*Kristallnacht*" (Night of the Broken Glass), a night of terror. Nazi soldiers torched synagogues. Broke windows. Bloodied people. Raped women.

BOB WELCH

For Jews such as the Slangers, the event was chillingly reminiscent of the *pogroms* in Poland. The zeppelin-sized shadow of Nazism was growing larger. In September 1939, the Slangers gathered round the Philco radio and listened to the chilling news of war. Hungry for land, thirsty to avenge its humiliation in World War I, and anxious to rid the world of Jews, Germany had unleashed a *Blitzkrieg* invasion of Poland on September 1, 1939, killing 50,000 civilians—equal to the population of Boston's entire South End. Warsaw was in ruins. In the city's most exclusive residential district, desperate people cut up dead horses to avoid starving to death. World War II had begun.

Already, Hitler had forged a secret deal with Russian leader Joseph Stalin to split Poland between the two countries. The eastern half became Soviet territory, the western half, German. The German plan was to make certain parts of Poland *Judenrein*. Jew-free. All Jews in Poland would be clustered into small areas, called ghettos, that would be reachable by rail. And one of those ghettos would be established in a city that, for all its bitter memories, was hidden deep in the soul of Frances Slanger: Lødz, the city where she'd been born. A week after entering Poland, German soldiers neared the city. "God, what's going on!" a fifteen-year-old Jewish boy from Lødz, Dawid Sierakowiak, wrote in his journal. "Panic, mass exodus . . . In the streets, crying, sobbing, wailing." Two days later, German soldiers swarmed into Lødz, Poland's second-largest city. They looted, torched homes, destroyed synagogues, and beat up Jews. Some Poles were more than happy to help. It surprised the Germans, for example, how willingly some would hold an Orthodox Jew while a soldier took a knife to his beard.

German soldiers raised a barbed-wire fence to enclose the 1.54-square-mile area that would form the ghetto. Growling dogs braced to spring on Jews who pushed the limits. Guards with machine guns stood ready to shoot if any made it to the fence. Edicts were soon posted, among them: "Jews are to wear a Jewish star, 10 centimeters high, on their right breast and back."

On April 30, 1940, the Lødz Ghetto, one of twelve such encampments to be established in Poland, was the first to be sealed, locking in 170,000 Jews, including dozens of Frances's relatives. Along with Jews brought in by train from other parts of Europe, the people were crammed, sometimes ten to a room, in tiny apartments. They were herded into factories, to help sustain the German war machine by helping to produce munitions. Some of the Lødz Jews would be worked to death. Thousands would die of disease and starvation. Others would die far quicker deaths—in places beyond.

In Normandy, Shoham left Frances to help prepare dinner. Frances went back on duty in the surgical tent. Capt. John Bonzer, the Y-tube of his stethoscope hanging from his neck, bent over a GI whose rib cage, X-rays would soon show, looked like a spilled game of pickup sticks.

"Need chest X-rays of this guy," he said.

"Right away, Johnny," said Frances, one of three nurses on duty. Technically, she was Schwartz's nurse—as perfectionists, they worked well together—but when something needed doing, protocol flew out the window.

For some reason, Frances always called Bonzer "Johnny," not that he minded. Frances was nobody's idea of a good time, but Bonzer liked her. She was mysterious, a loner, at times aloof, but he'd come to understand why: It was, he believed, because everything seemed to mean more to her than to the others. And he honored such perspective, even if all he wanted to do was get this war over and get back home—to some hospital where you didn't have to drop your scalpel into a disinfectant container fashioned from a C-ration can.

At the other end of the tent, Maj. Herman Lord, clamp in hand, tried to patch a sucking-chest wound. It was among the more common wounds seen in a field hospital. It tore open ribs and the sternum, often puncturing the lungs. The sucking sound came as the injured man gasped for breath, not from his mouth but from his chest.

Herman McNeill Lord was the commanding officer of the seventy-five person Second Platoon. He was a doctor from Detroit. He wore wire-rim glasses, sported a thin mustache, and occasionally—he hated wearing the things—donned a helmet that tilted on his head at an angle, as if his head simply weren't meant to be wearing it. The son of a minister, he had a wife back home named Wilma. He seemed far too frumpy to be a major. And yet he was no draftee like most of the rest. He'd enlisted in January 1940, four years after graduating from Wayne Medical College in Detroit. He did his job, was good with a scalpel— "one swell surgeon," in the eyes of one staff sergeant—and, though no battle-hardened leader, triggered few complaints from the men and women of the Second.

In the dank, cave-like tents, Frances and the other nurses hustled from shock to X-ray to surgery to post-op. They boiled glass syringes to sterilize them, adjusted oxygen masks, took temperatures, and gave shots of penicillin. To give shots—perhaps fifty in a session—one nurse loaded the syringe and changed needles, the other two gave the hypos. It was challenging enough during the day, more so at night when nurses were going between tents anchored by spiderwebs of ropes and pegs. And challenging enough dealing with soldiers, all the more when French civilians and an occasional German solider were added to the mix. ("Civilian male, boy, admitted with comminuted fracture of skull . . . in convulsions . . . transferred from 42nd Field Hospital . . . lingered 10 hours with progressive failure. Cause of death: comminuted fracture of skull . . . Civilian boy: booby trap

casualty . . . Shock severe. Cause of death: pulmonary edema secondary to anesthesia . . . Civilian adult female: admitted at full
term pregnancy . . . Delivers stillborn child . . . patient expired
0605 hours . . . Cause of death: parturition.")

Most surgeries—fifty to one hundred in a given day—were
done by Third Auxiliary doctors, who'd been attached to the
Forty-fifth Field Hospital since soon after Slanger's unit came
ashore. Rookie doctors, among them Bonzer and Schwartz,
assisted. Forty-fifth nurses only rarely dealt with actual surgeries. They did, however, do seemingly everything else on their
twelve-hour shifts, from monitoring vitals to changing dressings
to holding hands—occasionally, during heavy antiaircraft fire,
while wearing three-pound helmets.

Boston City this was not, Frances soon realized.
Generator-run lights hung from aluminum tent poles, offering a
weak, almost brown glow that funneled through lamp shades
fashioned from five-gallon tin cans. Rubber surgical gloves, dry-
ing after being sanitized, hung on makeshift clotheslines. Bedpan
covers had been made from parachute silk. Fly traps were
propped here and there. Bandages, for quick access, hung from
the tent's ceilings like tattered prom decorations. Coffee cups
and cigarette butts littered the nonsurgical areas.

The surgical tent, with six tables, offered relative opulence:
a white canvas floor, white walls, and white mosquito netting. In
other areas of the field hospital, boots quickly turned grass walk-
ways to mud. No privacy curtains protected a soldier's pride. A
field hospital was an open book where physical and emotional
pain was laid bare for all to see. Still, doctors, nurses, and the
wounded treated each other with a reverence—even if occasionally laced with black humor—that would seem unlikely in such a
horrific setting.

By now, Bonzer had moved on to another case: helping a
Third Auxiliary surgeon get some gut-shot soldier to his twenty-

first birthday. Frances was dabbing the soldier's forehead with a wet towel. Suddenly, a private rushed into the tent and said something to Major Lord, who'd just finished his surgery. Lord ripped off his rubber gloves and clapped his hands.

"Let's go!" said Lord. "We're movin' to Fauville. Jerry's headin' this way."

"Son of a bitch!" blistered the usually good-humored Bonzer. Groans rippled across the camp. Rookies such as Bonzer and Hirsh, who'd both gone to Temple University Medical School in Philadelphia, and Schwartz, who'd gone to Tufts Medical School in Boston, had been thrown into assisting on levels of surgeries that they'd never encountered. Stateside emergency rooms hadn't offered anything like the wounds made by high-velocity missiles. Bonzer's internship before the war, in Thomasville, Georgia, hadn't exactly helped. He'd spent much of it sprawled poolside at a guest plantation. Now all he and the other docs had to do was save lives while German soldiers were bearing down on them and nurses were packing their equipment for another move, their third in five days.

Frances hustled to her tent to get her gear. Across the way, Shoham, ever the chronicler, pulled a notebook from his pocket and quickly jotted "15 June: Moved to Fauville" just below "11 June: Moved to Audoville la Hubert." Then he stuffed it back into his pocket and hurried into the mess tent to get the kitchen packed.

"Wait a minute," said one of his cooks. "Ain't Fauville the place we just came from 'fore here?"

"Welcome to the army, Reb," said Shoham.

CHAPTER 6

*Be thou with the afflicted who flee away from the cruelty of
the oppressor. Quench the passions of fanaticism and
hatred . . .*

—FROM "PRAYER FOR THE JEWS OF RUSSIA,"
FOUND IN FRANCES SLANGER'S CHAPBOOK

Frances Slanger and the nurses in the Second Platoon got the
routine down quickly: first, when looking for a place to set
up the tents, look for a field with grazing cows. A field with dead
cows often meant a field littered with land mines.

Second, never head to the latrine without an enlisted man
to guard against the German prisoners of war who weren't to be
alone around nurses—and preferably make it an enlisted man
more interested in your safety than your feminine allure. Nurses,
as officers, were off-limits to enlisted men, but that didn't keep
some of them from taking their chances. The slit-trench latrines
of the first few days had been replaced by portable wooden priv-
ies, four-holers surrounded by canvas tarps. "Finally," Sallylou
told Dottie, "a use for our gas masks."

Third, never use an unsanitized catheter on a patient that
some dimwit private has been carrying around in a field jacket
pocket for a couple of days as if it were nothing more than a ball-
point pen.

Fourth, if stymied for a particular tool, use your helmet; one nurse had found twenty-one uses for the steel pot, from mixing bowl to bathtub to sitting stool.

And, finally, know the location of the nearest foxhole for when the German planes might drop their next batch of eggs; otherwise the preceding four points might be moot.

At night, unless it was blanketed by heavy cloud cover, the Normandy sky lit up with sound and fury as *Luftwaffe* aircraft swung over with their "bed-check Charlies." Blackouts were enforced. Smoking had to be done inside tents where men— nurses smoked rarely, and, if then, secretly—puffed mightily on cigarettes, cigars, and pipes.

Once, when John's Second Platoon and Sallylou's First Platoon had rendezvoused, the two were reacquainting themselves in a foxhole when a shell landed nearby. The explosion rained down dirt—even a little shrapnel—that sprinkled the two like rice thrown on church-fleeing newlyweds.

Already, the two missed the carefree days of England, when the Forty-fifth had been billeted in Upton-on-Severn. In bicycle rides across the English countryside and on evenings in front of fires upstairs in Upton's Odd Fellows Hall, the two had, if not fallen in love, at least conveniently forgotten that they were "attached" to others back home. Sallylou thought John was handsome, brilliant, and "bookish." It didn't hurt that he had the rosiest cheeks she'd ever seen and smoked a pipe with Wilkie tobacco, her favorite. John thought Sallylou was beautiful, confident, and slightly dangerous—in the best of senses. In many ways, the two were polar opposites, she as vivacious as he was reserved. But they clicked. Though both had others back home, the trip across the Atlantic, the country roads of England, and daily doses of wounded soldiers made home grow so small that at times they almost forgot what it was.

When John, Sallylou, and others from the Forty-fifth had

gathered in Upton for drinks in the evenings at a pub below the Odd Fellows Hall, though, Frances wasn't there. Nor when groups would ride through the English countryside, their journeys sometimes turning into "pub crawls" from one country watering hole to the next and occasionally leading to what was known in wartime England as the "3B fracture: beer, blackout, and bicycle."

For some reason, Frances had been the lone nurse billeted by herself in Upton. Thinking her lonely, Ed Bowen and Monty—the two who'd become engaged on their last night before shipping out of New York—occasionally visited her in her room. But Frances hadn't become a total hermit. She'd gone into London with others on a two-day pass and was occasionally seen walking on the riverbank with a tall doctor, Isadore Schwartz.

Despite their size difference, the two had much in common. Both were Jewish, had grown up within ten miles of each other, and had fathers who had been fruit peddlers. Both were deeply committed to their patients. When Schwartz was an intern at Charles V. Chapin Hospital in Providence, Rhode Island, Monty had watched him save a child's life—on a night he wasn't even supposed to be on duty. Both could muster humor when necessary; Schwartz loved a good priest/rabbi joke, and Frances's writing was sprinkled with levity. But, for the most part, the two were serious-minded perfectionists about their medical roles, specifically about helping people get better. Sometimes they were so serious that they ran afoul of those who didn't seem to care as much as they did.

From a distance, a few wondered if they'd become lovers, but those who knew them well—Schwartz's tent mate, Shoham, for example—thought otherwise. Schwartz was a married man and, though some officers weren't about to let that get in the way of an affair, Frances respected such boundaries. If war had a way of making some men and women forget about promised ones back home—John and Sallylou quickly did—it didn't do so for Isadore Schwartz. He and Frances, whether working together on a patient or sharing a cup of coffee in the mess tent, seemed connected by something—something deep—but it wasn't romance. It was, believed some, something beyond.

ONE NIGHT, all was quiet, or as quiet as Normandy ever got on a cloud-free night when planes were buzzing overhead. The three platoons of the Forty-fifth were bivouacked together somewhere on the Contentin Peninsula. Who knew where anymore? Night-shift personnel tended the wounded. Day-shift personnel, in darkened tents, lay awake, wondering how much more of this they could take, or slept, dreaming of home or loved ones or Ingrid Bergman or Frankie Sinatra, the new female heartthrob who—

Suddenly, gunfire shattered the slumber. Not just single shots. But rapid-fire bursts, as if from a machine gun. People awoke, disoriented, hearts pounding. Instinctively, they slid outside the tents and skittered into foxholes. The gunfire kept popping . . . then slowed . . . became more sporadic . . . and, finally, died out. The Forty-fifth's camp lay frozen in fear. Finally, a few voices arose near the camp's dump sight. The exchange grew louder—and finally the voice of a sleep-shattered captain thundered in the night.

"Who's the jackass who didn't check for ammo in the pockets before burning the uniforms?"

FRANCES SLANGER and the other nurses slept in sixteen-foot-by-sixteen-foot cotton-duck tents that, like the rest, were olive green and water repellent, but not waterproof. In this abnormally wet June, roofs sometimes sagged like bulging water balloons. Nurses who accidentally brushed against them would trigger drips that could go on for days. The tents had no floors. Tables fashioned from wooden bomb crates and four cots comprised the furniture. Virtually everything inside was bathed in a monochrome of khaki except for white and pink brassieres and panties strung on laundry lines.

The medical tents were far larger than the officers' quarters. They were four-peaked and rectangular, humped at the tent poles like the saddle sweep of circus tents: one pre-op ("shock") tent, one surgical, and one post-op, linked together like a train. These were flanked by nearly a dozen other large tents, among them pharmacy, supply, X-ray, headquarters, and Captain Shoham's love-it-or-leave-it mess hall. On the camp's edges, the humble pup tents of enlisted men popped up at each location like tidily placed green houses in a Monopoly game. The Platoon's "village" covered an area about the size of a large city block.

Frances's Second Platoon "bunkies," or tent mates, were three nurses also from Massachusetts: Christine Cox, Margaret Bowler, and Elizabeth Powers. Cox, twenty-three, was the lanky, green-eyed daughter of Irish immigrants and had grown up in blue-blooded Prides Crossing, north of Boston. She arrived at Fort Devens two weeks before Frances, bringing with her a nursing degree from Massachusetts General Hospital, an appreciation for good poetry, and a keen sense of humor. She lacked the mischievousness of a Sallylou Cummings, the student nurse who'd once dressed up a school skeleton in a nursing cape to mock a particularly ornery teacher—and nearly had her graduation privileges revoked because of it. But Cox nevertheless leavened her tent with a lighter touch. And liked Frances Slanger. Back at Fort Devens, when Frances's autograph book had asked for "Service addresses," Cox had written, "Wherever you go, kid." Christine couldn't resist a barb. "To a good little 'gold britches,' " she wrote. " 'What, are you off duty again???' I'm only kidding, honey."

Margaret Bowler, thirty-three, was also Irish. She'd grown up in Westfield, Massachusetts, a boilermaker's daughter who'd witnessed death up close long before entering the service. Two of her sisters had died when they were young, callousing Margaret to the world at large. Like Frances, she'd had a caregiver's heart since she was young. Once, when a niece took sick, Margaret had insisted the little girl come stay with Margaret and her family. "Don't worry," she said. "I'm going to take care of you."

Elizabeth Powers had grown up in Lowell, Massachusetts. At thirty-four, she was one of the Second's older, and more serious, nurses—a "biddy" in the eyes of some. She aggravated Capain Shoham no end with her special-order meal requests for patients. *What did she think this was? The Waldorf-Astoria?*

The four women, all brunettes, may not have made for the most raucous tent, but they certainly were the most ecumenical: two Catholics (Bowler and Powers), a Protestant (Cox), and a Jew (Slanger). The four had grown to know each other well, having been together since their basic-training days at Fort Devens. That's where Frances Slanger's war had begun: at a camp about forty miles northwest of Boston, near Ayer, Massachusetts, in August 1943. It took Frances, with friend Jack Goodman at the wheel, about ninety minutes to get there. But, in some ways, it took years.

SHE WAS a young woman, roughly the same age as Frances, and had been admitted to Boston City Hospital on June 24, 1941, a day when passengers on the elevated trains were absorbed in front-page stories about German troops having now invaded the Soviet Union—and slaughtering civilians along the way.

The woman, married with two young children, was a patient of Frances's, and was dying. She had cancer, a tumor on her pituitary gland. Doctors gave her only weeks to live. After the woman had undergone surgery, Frances took her blood pressure every day, her pulse every half hour, her respiration every fifteen minutes. She soaked a sponge in tepid alcohol and dabbed the woman's face to help ease an elevated temperature. She helped doctors give her daily—sometimes twice daily—blood transfusions. And yet on the twelfth day, the woman died.

As a nurse, Frances was becoming more familiar with death. But this woman's death moved Frances in a way the others had not. It wasn't only that she'd watched the woman's husband and two children visit every day for two weeks. It was that this single, antiseptic, middle-class Catholic death in Boston, Massachusetts, had stirred in Frances the wider reality of thousands of grittier deaths an ocean away. War deaths. Not only of soldiers, but of civilians, the innocent bystanders who found themselves in the way of men fighting each other. The civilians in Poland. Now the civilians in the Soviet Union. Unlike most others, she understood the plight of such people. After all, she'd once been one.

The night before the Fourth of July, as firecrackers from early-bird revelers popped in the distance, Frances sat behind her typewriter and began to write:

> She had received every last rite from the priest—and daily Masses were being held for her. Everything that was humanly and scientifically possible was being done to save her for a husband who worshipped her and two adoring children. She had everything to live for.
>
> I can't help but marvel at the idiosyncrasies of life. Under this same sun, moon, and stars, on another part of this planet, wholesale murder, wholesale slaughter of

innocent women and children is taking place. Men have to go out to kill and be killed. Why? There is no priest, minister or rabbi to comfort the wounded and administer last rites to the dying. The discoveries of science are used to destroy and not to help civilization. In many cases, there is no one around to stop a hemorrhage, ease pain, or give a drink of water to fever-parched lips.

Here we work so hard to save one life; *there* they work so hard to end life. It just doesn't make sense: beautiful landscapes, the exquisite work of architects, poets, authors, and artists is annihilated, perhaps never to be replaced again.

At last my patient is pronounced dead. Yet even in death I cannot help but think how much more fortunate she is than millions of other human beings elsewhere. I keep asking myself: Why? Why? Why? There is no answer.

When my head touches my pillow at night, I fervently thank God that I am living in these United States of America. I thank God that in our way we *save* life. And I pray that our beautiful flag will continue to wave over the land of the free and the home of the brave.

As the summer of 1941 deepened, so, too, did Frances's sense that the world was made up of haves and have-nots. And she knew exactly where she fit. Had her family not escaped Poland when it did, before America instituted the 1921 Quota Law that drastically curtailed immigration, the Slangers almost certainly would be locked in the Lødz Ghetto right now, among the "have-nots." Just like her relatives were. As it was, she felt soothed by a certain sense of privilege, though it was now becoming a worrisome privilege.

Guilt? A lack of response toward the evil in the world?

Who knew what was stirring Frances Slanger's soul. But in the summer of 1941, two things moved her: One was the death of the young mother as the Germans invaded the Soviet Union. The other was the realization that the U.S. Army, with the possibility of war for America creeping closer, was seeking nurses.

Evil, she realized, was loose in the world. The call for nurses offered her a way to help counter that evil, if even in a small way. America's isolationist freeze was thawing. If the country wasn't at war, it was clearly preparing for it. And, in some ways, so was Frances Slanger.

As GERMANY invaded the Soviet Union, it used special mobile killing squads called *Einsatzgruppen* to kill Jews. The civilians would be taken outside of town, forced to dig their own graves, stripped, then shot. Children watched their parents die in a tangle of bodies, bullet holes in their necks. Parents watched their children die the same way. From June 1941 to December 1941, the *Einsatzgruppen* killed nearly half a million Jews.

Now, though, German leaders came to believe that the approach lacked efficiency and was overly stressful on those doing the shooting. Starvation in ghettos such as Lødz was having a minimal impact, particularly with Jewish women still having babies. Suicides helped, of course; in Lødz, Jews killed themselves by a number of methods, from jumping out windows to eating matchsticks to hanging themselves. But such deaths, the Germans realized, weren't effective enough, given the masses of Jews still alive.

They came to realize something else was required, a "final solution."

In 1941, as summer's heat sent Boston's elite packing for the ocean-cooled beaches at Ipswich and Smith's Point and Beverly

Manchester Cove, Frances Slanger's life had become gnarled like never before. The previous November, David had had a stroke that left him partially paralyzed; he had been placed in Jewish Memorial Hospital with little hope of ever leaving it. Overnight, Frances suddenly became the family breadwinner. And now the war was growing closer to her.

The little girl who'd grown up with World War I raging on her doorstep now lamented what relatives in Lødz must be experiencing. Frances's poetry, once glittered with a sort of Dale Carnegie optimism, was tainted with fatalism. She looked in the newspapers and saw a world turning darker. She looked in the mirror and saw a twenty-eight-year-old woman who'd gained some weight and whose dreams had blown away; gone were the days of lounging on a sofa at a Cape Cod summer cottage, lost in a book. In one poem, she suggested that her life was mired in meaninglessness.

I have lived my life in vain
Now I see past years drift by
And my heart is full of pain
For I am about to die.

America was edging closer toward war. The need for nurses beckoned from the posters and the pages of *Life* magazine and from the newspaper columns, radio talks, and speeches by First Lady Eleanor Roosevelt. "We need 200,000 nurses' aides," she said in a talk at the Brooklyn Jewish Center that made national news. "The Red Cross can train only 3,000 every seven weeks, and we may find this shortage a very serious one as the needs of the armed forces increase." Frances's restlessness surged. Perhaps she should join the U.S. Army Nurse Corps.

Her parents hardly encouraged such thinking. Though patriotic to their cores, they were steeped in a Jewish tradition that discouraged the slightest risk for women. What's more, they were dependent on her. She was making $100 a month at the hospital; could she make that kind of money in the army?

Frances's caregiver bent had worn such a deep groove in her life that even the thought of straying from it triggered guilt. Caregivers hate to cause others pain. They live to *ease* others' pain. When Frances considered leaving, she was haunted by the same thought she'd had when walking into Boston City Hospital to inquire about nursing school: *traitor.*

She also abhorred the idea of leaving her nephews, five-year-old Irwin and nearly one-year-old Jerry. She'd once written a lighthearted poem about Irwin, pretending she was referring to the man of her dreams, then ending it: "He's all I've wanted him to be/I would not change his weight for gold/Alas, how fast the days go by/For soon he'll be two years old!" To Sally's sons, Aunt Frances had become a fairy godmother in pedal pushers. She climbed with the boys in the neighbor's chestnut tree on Homestead Street in Roxbury, where the family had recently moved to a bow-faced apartment. She took them to Franklin Park and rode the merry-go-round with them. She wrote poems about them, read them books, and sang them to sleep. At night, saying her prayers, she literally thanked God for the two boys— even if they sometimes ran her ragged.

But amid such pulls to stay, Frances craved adventure. Life at home, she wrote, had become "dull and boring." And deeper things pulled. In October 1941, President Franklin Roosevelt set in motion the first peacetime draft in U.S. history. Hundreds of thousands of new soldiers and sailors poured into basic training at camps that had sprung up across the country like spring weeds. At Fort Bragg, in North Carolina, barracks sprouted at the rate of one building every thirty-two minutes, with 700 southern lumber mills working overtime to keep up with the demand.

The majority of men who began occupying those barracks weren't there by choice; they'd been drafted. But one late-summer day, in the boldest decision she'd made since entering nursing school eight years before, Frances Slanger chose to join the U.S. Army Nurse Corps. Not because the law required it. But because she thought it was simply the right thing to do. And because with each article she pasted into her chapbook about the Germans' treatment of the Jews, Frances could imagine what it must be like for an aunt, an uncle, or a cousin back in Poland.

In Lødz, a young woman and her four-year-old daughter, blue-eyed and blond, were taken out to the courtyard for "selection." The woman's husband, a doctor, had already been shot while try-ing to escape. She held her daughter by the hand. The girl must be taken, a German officer told her. The mother smiled and would not let go of her daughter's hand. Did she really intend to resist? Yes, the mother said, continuing to smile. The man was different from other officers, the woman realized. Compassion-ate. He gave her a three-minute stay, then asked if she still in-tended to resist. Yes, she said, still smiling. The compassion drained from the soldier's face. Turn to the wall, he commanded. He then fired bullets into the heads of both mother and daughter.

Meanwhile, in the fall of 1941, experiments by the Germans showed that an ordinary pesticide called Zyklon B—originally developed for exterminating household pests—could be used to kill human beings. The pellets, like rock salt, could be poured into showers or other chambers from openings in the roofs, releasing a deadly gas. The people below would be dead within twenty minutes. Death could be accomplished much more efficiently than shooting or another method the Germans had begun using to kill Jews: piping exhaust fumes into vans stuffed with people. The new method, they believed, was a far better "final solution."

Camps would be built in Poland, the location chosen because of it having the highest concentration of Jews in Europe and it being relatively isolated. Then, Jews from all over Europe could be brought by rail to these places. The new setups would be called "reeducation camps."

THE ARMY instructed Frances to report to a camp of her own on or about November 12, 1941: Lovell General Hospital at Fort Devens. "Sufficient notice will be given to enable you to arrange your personal affairs," Ruth Taylor, an assistant supervisor with the Army Nurse Corps, wrote to Frances.

But some "personal affairs," Frances discovered, aren't easily arranged. In early October, Frances's father had a second stroke. By now, she had gotten used to the idea of her new adventure, of leaving home, of taking action on the patriotism she had only effused in prose and poetry. But with news of her father's worsening condition, any belief that she actually *deserved* to leave home fell away amid her sense of responsibility. At sixty, her father might be near death. How could she leave him now? She had only one choice: She notified the army of her decision to rescind her enlistment.

"We are very sorry to hear of your father's illness and will be glad to talk over ways and means with you anytime you can come to this office," wrote the ANC's Taylor. "We will put your application in the deferred file."

Deferred. For Frances Slanger, it had a familiar ring to it.

AS SHE WAITED, so, too, did the Jews of Lødz. But when Japan's bombing of Pearl Harbor drew the United States into World

War II in December 1941, the Jews rejoiced. By now, six death camps had been established, all within 200 miles of the city. Rail lines directly linked Lødz to Auschwitz to the south and Chelmno to the east; most Lødz Jews would die in these two camps. But now came a flicker of hope for liberation; perhaps the Americans would be the saviors of the Jews.

The war, however, began badly for America. On March 11, 1942, with the Japanese capture of the island of Corregidor imminent, Gen. Douglas MacArthur was forced to leave the Philippines. MacArthur was distraught, leaving behind nearly 80,000 troops who would die or be forced to surrender, then likely tortured. When he arrived in Darwin, Australia, MacArthur made what would become an historic promise: "I came through," he wrote on the back of an envelope, and handed to Australian reporters, "and I shall return!"

Two weeks later, 999 Jews from Slovakia made history, too. They comprised the first trainload of Jews to depart for Auschwitz in the darkness of cattle cars. Unlike MacArthur, they would not return.

On June 26, 1942, the *Boston Globe* became one of the first U.S. papers to report the atrocities against the Jews. "Mass Murders of Jews in Poland Pass 700,000," read a headline on a story relegated, oddly, to the bottom of page 12. Such news brought to mind for Frances the dim memories of aunts and uncles and cousins who'd been with her in Lødz. Where were they now?

U.S. president Franklin Roosevelt and British prime minister Winston Churchill vowed to hold the Nazis responsible for the murders of Jews, but still considered the "Jewish problem" a secondary issue to the war itself. They believed the best way to save the Jews was to win the war. As news spread of the planned Allied invasion of France—and the condition of her father improved—Frances reconsidered the idea of joining the Army

Nurse Corps. Soon, she realized, American soldiers would be battling the same German forces that were holding her relatives prisoner in Lødz, that were, as she'd written, responsible for the "wholesale slaughter of innocent women and children." And, if so, who would be there to help "stop a hemorrhage, ease pain, or give a drink of water to fever-parched lips . . . ?"

As Frances weighed her future, First Lady Eleanor Roosevelt continued to urge young women to consider military nursing. "You must not forget," she said in one of her many radio pep talks to nurses, "that you have it in your power to bring back some who otherwise surely will not return."

In downtown Boston, a passing band struck up a spirited rendition of "The Stars and Stripes Forever" as part of the Armistice Day parade on November 11, 1942. Frances watched from the throngs lining the streets, honoring the World War I soldiers who'd been to war—and the World War II soldiers who would soon be leaving—as they marched by.

Afterward, she walked to the nearby Boston Public Gardens, where she'd heard a floral portrait had been created to honor her hero, General MacArthur. Part of the display was his "I will return" promise. She found it amid the park's gardens, pond, and statues—and was so moved that she wrote a poem about it:

I gazed for a long time.
And as I edged away
The inscription singed itself into my soul,
And I felt
That his promise would be fulfilled!
He will return—
In children's laughter:

In the silver resonance of church bells on Sunday:
In the quiet of classrooms:
In the turbulence of factories:
In the peace of gardens:
In the satisfaction of individual achievements.
He will return
In all things dear to free people.

MacArthur would seem an unlikely hero for Frances Slanger. The two could not have been more different: he a gentile male general with an ego so large that his press officers had to alter publicity releases if he wasn't sufficiently ballyhooed; she an obscure Jewish female nurse with an inferiority complex. But she revered the man. He gave her hope. He had been turned back, defeated, deterred—she knew the feeling well—but had vowed to return. Might she, too?

As the last of Roxbury's autumn leaves fell and winter began bullying New England, Frances continued to mull her future. Everywhere, soldiers were saying good-byes. One of her few friends, a soda jerk who made her chocolate malted milks at The Corner Drug near the Northampton Elevated Station, had left for the navy. Nathan Fleishman was heartened at how consistently Frances wrote—"I always knew I could depend on you," he wrote back—and anxiously awaited word that she might join the Army Nurse Corps. But a postcard from Frances contained no such news; instead, it was almost entirely about a sick patient of hers who she was worried about.

By now, Frances had become a private-duty nurse in individual homes, because it paid more and meant freedom from hovering "snoopervisors." And with her father's health improving, she revisited the idea of enlisting. But if, in the last two years, the parental front warmed to the military idea, a cultural cold front had replaced it. Though women were, in 1943, being allowed into Harvard classrooms for the first time, support for women serving in the military was thin at best.

Still, the atrocities in Europe kept tugging at Frances. In her chapbook, Frances pasted "The Murder of Lidice," a lengthy poem she'd found in the October 19, 1942, issue of *Life* magazine. It was written by Pulitzer Prize–winning poet Edna St. Vincent Millay about Lidice, a small, predominantly Jewish village in Czechoslovakia where the Germans, on June 10, 1942, had executed 246 adults and deported dozens of women and children to concentration camps. In one part of a lengthy poem, Millay wrote of a young Jewish mother who, with the Germans pounding on her door, hid her newborn baby under a bed.

> "There's nobody here but me," she said;
> And her eyes were bright and hot in her head.
> "I'm far too sick of the fever," she said,
> "Into Germany, into Germany,
> For to be marched or led!"
> But the baby wailed from under the bed—
> And they by the heels with a harsh shout
> Did drag him out . . . but the baby bled—
> So against the wall they banged his head,
> While the mother clawed at their clothes and screamed,
> And screamed, and screamed till they shot her dead.

On May 2, 1943, a Sunday afternoon, more than 20,000 people gathered in Boston Gardens to protest German atrocities against the Jews. It was believed to be the greatest mass meeting in the history of New England. Meanwhile, the nationwide call for nurses intensified. "This is our hour—the hour toward which everything in our past lives has been leading," Maj. Julia C. Stimson of the Army Nurse Corps had written for the *American*

Journal of Nursing, a magazine Frances read regularly. "We cannot deny the fact that the war can be lost. If we and others refuse to believe this and remain careless of our country's danger, the fate of other unprepared peoples can be ours. But now the time of excuses and delays is past."

Frances Slanger apparently agreed. In the spring of 1943, she joined the Army Nurse Corps, this time for good. Soon she would be headed for Europe to help Allied forces stop the Nazis' choke hold on the world.

Frances underwent a physical examination on June 5, 1943, at the Army Service Forces' personnel headquarters in downtown Boston. Two weeks later, a letter arrived in the mail on Homestead Street in Roxbury. Frances hurriedly skimmed the words from 1st Lt. Katherine F. Mullane of the Army Nurse Corps: "Dear Miss Slanger . . . given a final-type physical . . . and that you have been found qualified . . ."—at last, she had been accepted!

But, wait, what was this? ". . . for limited military service with a waiver of defective vision, bilateral." In other words, poor eyesight in both eyes.

"*Limited* military service?"

Frances read on. "The present policy as pertains to a nurse found qualified for limited military service means that she may be assigned to duty within the continental limits of the United States. She is not qualified, however, for transfer to foreign service."

Frances slumped into a chair. *Not qualified for overseas duty?*

She was to report to Fort Devens on or about July 15. From there, who knew where she was headed—apparently not Europe, which now raised a question in her mind: Should she proceed with her enlistment or, with no apparent chance to serve overseas, simply walk away?

Frances signed the papers. "Defective" or not, she would enlist. She would prove she was good enough. She would find a way to go where she knew she needed to be.

• • •

WHEN AUNT FRANCES walked down the street, her two nephews thought the world lit up around her like fairy dust. But now she was walking away from them—from Irwin, from Jerry, from her family, from Roxbury. On a hot, humid Monday, August 2, 1943, Frances said her good-byes. She was headed for Fort Devens and a first-of-its-kind basic training program for nurses.

If, in saying good-bye, Eva and David worried about their daughter's safety, it wasn't because newspapers, magazines, and radio had been recounting the daily carnage of war. The government prohibited releasing photos of American dead for the first part of the war; not until a month after Frances left for Fort Devens, ironically, would the government loosen its restrictions. Still, the Slangers knew enough about war—and had read enough casualty lists in the papers—to know some soldiers get wounded, some die, and some get captured. And nurses weren't exempt. The Slangers surely had heard about Dorothy C. Morse, Boston City Hospital School of Nursing Class of '39, who had died when the Red Cross ship she was on en route to England had been torpedoed by a German U-boat. And had probably heard about the nurses who'd been captured by the Japanese in the Philippines.

First, Frances said good-bye to her mother, who was now sixty-one. Eva Slanger's face was strained by time and by David's hospitalization, but the woman remained Frances's rock of stability. The two hugged long and hard. She said good-bye to her father at Jewish Memorial Hospital, the parting made more poignant by the realization that she might never see him again. As a nurse, she knew he was slowly dying. As a daughter, she didn't want to believe it. She leaned over him, as he lay in bed, and hugged him one last time.

The good-bye with her sister and nephews came in Hull, a blue-collar beach community on a finger of land that jutted into the Atlantic Ocean southeast of Boston. James and Sally and the

BOB WELCH

boys lived in a three-story bungalow just east of the corner of
Warren and Nantasket, about a block from where the Atlantic
rolled ashore.

At nearby Pemberton Point, neckers—many of them soldiers and their girls—gathered each evening for passion and
good-bye promises, few of which would be kept. And across
Hingham Bay to the west, the Quincy shipyard continued its
nonstop drive to build ships for the invasion of Europe.

On this sweltering summer day, Frances stood on the beach
at Hull and breathed deep the salt air. Waves folded neatly from
blue to white. Seagulls squawked. A little boy stood in the
Atlantic, tugging a toy sailboat back and forth on a string. It was
Irwin, her seven-year-old nephew. Time and again, he would let
out the boat and time and again it would crash awkwardly
ashore, languishing at the whim of the waves.

The two walked back to the house, an off-white, Cape-style
home with an open porch on front. Frances patted a spot on the
swing next to her. She put her arm around him and he lay his
head in her lap. Then she began singing him "Brahms Lullaby,"
his favorite song: "Lullaby and good night, with roses
bedight/With lilies o'er spread is baby's wee bed. . . ."

Once finished, she told him she had to go away.

But *why?* He didn't understand. She told him it was just
something she needed to do.

But *why?* She was going to be a nurse in the army and take
care of the soldiers who would get hurt.

But *why?* He cried. That made her cry. She kissed him on
the cheek.

A family friend, Jack Goodman, rolled up in a car and put
Frances's two suitcases in the trunk. Frances gave Irwin one final
hug, then walked away. Irwin watched as the car headed south
down Nantucket Road and grew smaller and smaller until it disappeared.

He never saw her again.

CHAPTER 7

Keep your heart free from hate, your mind from worry. Live simply; expect little; give much; sing often; pray always. Fill your life with love; scatter sunshine. Forget self. Think of others. Do as you would be done by. These are the tried links in contentment's golden chain.

—McLeod,
found in Frances Slanger's chapbook

He was some kid from Tennessee who'd stumbled upon a nest of Germans dug into a hedgerow and wound up with a bellyful of lead. Near a village called Beuzeville au Plain, just west of Ste.-Mère-Église, Frances Slanger swathed his wound with a bandage. A light rain ushered in the growing twilight.

In the shock ward, there was no time to undress a GI or even take off his mud-caked boots. Frances swabbed the skin on his arm and injected a needle for an intravenous line. Soon, plasma flowed through his veins, gradually bringing color back to his face. A few cots down, a soldier moaned, some of his intestines still back in some unpronounceable French village. Next to him a buddy who'd taken a single bullet to the spine stared into nothingness, languid eyes locked in terror.

The shock ward was affectionately known as "The Chamber of Horrors." It was here where soldiers in shock needed to be revived enough so they could withstand surgery, here where life and death struggled with each other in hand-to-hand combat. Some soldiers arrived with their weapons virtually glued to them by mud and blood. Paper tags detailed their injuries and indicated how much morphine they had been given—"not enough," most of the wounded believed. Most soldiers were unconscious. All were helpless. They lay on cots—sixteen aligned on each side of the tent's outer edges, alternating directions so one man wouldn't be as apt to spread germs to another. They were covered with olive-drab woolen blankets. IVs hung above them like the barrage balloons back in the Bay of the Seine, the bottles of plasma dripping life into their outstretched arms.

In a connecting tent, where the surgical unit was cordoned off by mosquito netting, the newly arrived Third Auxiliary doctors operated on soldiers who had been placed on litters elevated by sawhorses. The Third's surgeons might have been notorious for taking dinner-line cuts, but nobody questioned their commitment to the soldiers. Once, a surgeon stayed all night with a wounded man in case the GI's catheter needed changing.

In the shock tent, where she spent much of her time, Frances checked the dressing of the kid from Tennessee. He was alive but listless.

"We'll get to him next," said Bonzer, taking a rare break from surgery to see what was coming. "He'll be ten pounds lighter when we get that shrapnel out of him."

Frances smiled self-consciously, then helped a patient get a rubber tube to his mouth for a sip of water. The tent smelled of sweat and smoke and excrement from torn bowels. It smelled of ether and mud and the occasional stomach-wrenching stench of gangrenous body parts, none of which seemed to dissuade Frances from being here. After all, she'd *fought* to be here.

Back home, the army's decision to keep her Stateside because of her poor eyesight had hung above her for months like a brooding cloud. As she'd gone through training at Fort Devens in Massachusetts, Fort Rucker in Alabama, and Camp Gordon in Georgia, it was as if she were doing all the homework like the other students in class but wasn't eligible for the year-end field trip. But the need for nurses, she knew, wasn't in the States; anyone could take blood pressures at a V.A. hospital. The need was overseas.

Frances had never been known for her *chutzpah*, nor did she have the kind of power to pull strings. But at some point during her training—probably during a seven-week stint at Camp Gordon in Georgia—she dared to question the Army Nurse Corps's decision to leave her home. Exactly when and how isn't known, but you can imagine a five-foot-one Jewish woman standing on one side of a desk and a grizzled male officer sitting on the other. The nervousness. The fear. The flashbacks to permission-seeking moments from decades long gone: permission to enter America, to start nursing school—"It's *not* for a Jewish girl!"—to join the U.S. Army Nurse Corps in the first place.

Now this: a plea to serve on the front lines in France. A plea to be in a position where, as the First Lady herself had implored, Frances and other nurses might help "bring back some who otherwise surely will not return." Soon, American soldiers would join their comrades who were now fighting in the South Pacific and North Africa by putting their lives on the line in France. And Frances Slanger believed she needed to be among them. Vision, she wanted to prove, had little to do with the eyes, and everything to do with the heart.

Whether it was the voracity of her argument or the ANC's realization that it was still short of nurses for an invasion against the most formidable army in the world, Frances Slanger won her case. She was given a waiver and cleared to serve where she wanted to serve: beside front-line soldiers.

• • •

"SOMEONE ORDER THESE?"

As rain drummed harder on the tent flap of the shock ward, the litter-bearers arrived with more wounded. They tried to keep things light when they'd arrive with another batch of patients; otherwise, they figured, they'd wind up in the shock ward themselves—with a thousand-yard stare of their own. That's why some named their jeeps such things as "Sudden Death," "Amen," or "You've Had It."

The wounded's journey here usually took an hour or two. From the point where a soldier was hit—some five to twenty miles away—a medic would sprinkle sulfa powder on the wound, slap a dressing on it, inject the man with morphine, and flag the litter-bearers to hustle him to the nearest jeep. From there he would go to a battalion aid station about 500 yards behind the front lines, then to a clearing station where triage doctors decided who could go directly to evac and who needed field-hospital surgery.

If the soldier had a serious stomach or chest wound, or was deep in shock from having lost a limb, he was sent to a field hospital. The moveable hospitals were the nearest completely equipped medical units to the fighting lines themselves.

The wounded arrived on stretchers, often buckled sideways four to a jeep—"like slaughtered deer," one such soldier quipped. Most would be deep in shock, having the metabolic rate of an old man, which often killed them before the effects of a wound itself.

With few exceptions, the Forty-fifth took "nontransportable" patients—those who would likely die if they didn't have immediate surgery. A field hospital was like a giant Intensive Care Unit. If a badly wounded soldier could undergo surgery within six hours of being hit, his survival rate was high. Those who lived—and the vast majority did—stayed with the unit for a week or two.

Then the soldiers were sent to a station hospital—a rear-echelon, semipermanent establishment, the last stop before a permanent hospital in England or the United States.

A soldier could be wounded in numerous ways. He could be peppered by shrapnel from a German 88, which fired twenty-two pound projectiles that traveled faster than the speed of sound. He could be shot with a vicious wooden bullet that splintered when it entered the body or stabbed in the gut while engaged in hand-to-hand combat in the parlor of some shell-strewn French villa. Like a young officer, and husband and father, just off Utah Beach, he could be walking beside an American tank in an enemy-safe area when the gunner in the turret accidentally gets thrown against his weapon, discharging it. And, just like that, a field hospital—or Graves Registration—had another customer. In rare cases, he could decide he'd had enough of this hell and shoot himself, usually in the left foot, in an attempt to get a ticket home—or a soldier could wind up in the 45th's tents for myriad other reasons.

Perforated guts, livers, spleens, kidneys, and lungs—Frances and the Second Platoon saw them all. The more dark-humored of field hospital personnel referred to their jobs as "graveyard salvage."

"Glad it's you in there and not me, *Hunzeczech,*" Shoham told Bonzer. "I'll stick to peeling potatoes and pulling teeth."

As a field hospital, the Forty-fifth's goal wasn't trying to make wounded soldiers "new again." Often, surgeons didn't even do sutures, leaving that for down-the-line docs without life-or-death patients on their stretchers. Instead, the goal for Bonzer, Schwartz, Hirsh, Lord, and the other Forty-fifth doctors was simple: to keep a man alive long enough so hospitals in the rear could put him back together again.

• • •

Elizabeth Powers, one of Frances's tent mates, bent closer to a wounded soldier to hear what his weary lips were uttering. His chest, heavily bandaged, rose and fell ever so slightly; he'd been burned when his tank had been hit.

"Where'd you say you were from again, soldier?" she asked.

"Asheville, ma'am . . . Asheville . . . North . . . Carolina."

They arrived, these wounded men, as strangers to the nurses. With roughly fifty patients spread throughout the tent village at any given time, the Forty-fifth had a smattering from dozens of states: a kid from Texas who'd been quarterbacking his high school football team a year before. A young man from Oregon whose wife was building ships in Portland. A teacher from Michigan hoping to be home by the time the school bells rang in September. But this one was from Asheville and Elizabeth immediately sent a private to hunt down Capt. Fred Michalove, who'd grown up there.

Michalove, who'd enlisted the day after the attack on Pearl Harbor, was the Second's chief administrative officer, the only officer in the unit who wasn't a doctor or a nurse. He was thirty-two, a slow-paced southerner who never made a decision without at least a couple of puffs on his pipe—quiet, thoughtful, and, by now, already weary of the ways of war. When he came to the soldier's side, he realized he didn't know him. But he talked to the wounded GI about how sweet the dogwoods in North Carolina smelled in the spring. How he used to sell hot dogs at Asheville Tourists minor league baseball games. And about working at the newspaper in town—how he'd interviewed a Nazi sympathizer for a story and told the guy, right up front, that he was Jewish. "And just to let you know," he said, "we know what your Hitler is up to."

By the time the conversation ended, it was hard to tell which man's eyes were mistier. Hearing such stories, Frances remembered the time before the war, in January 1941, when she'd walked into a corner room on Boston City's second floor to check on a patient. There, in an adjacent bed, was someone familiar: Milton Zola, whose father had worked the fruit route with Frances's father. He was eighteen and had just undergone emergency surgery for an appendectomy. Whatever nursing care he was getting, she decided, wasn't good enough.

"*Motle*," she said as Zola woke from a sleep. "It is me, *Faigie*. I am here for you."

Zola had been surprised to see Frances because his family had moved south to Dorchester in 1934. He hadn't seen her in years. She bent over him in her nurse whites. She treated him as if he were some sort of visiting dignitary and it was her responsibility to make him as comfortable as possible.

He wasn't her patient—she was taking care of three others in the room—but she made him her patient. He ate better than the others. He got attention faster than the others. He got more back rubs than the others. She was doing it not because he was her friend or because he was Jewish, Zola realized, but because she cared. He would never forget the gesture, small though it may have been. Not even when he, too, wound up in France as a solider playing this deadly game of war. Now, amid the human trauma in these tents, Frances greeted soldiers with the same gentle touch—as if the two were long lost friends. *It is me . . . I am here for you.* As if these soldiers were Milton Zola or the women and children of Eastern Europe she'd written about.

Joseph Shoham, who was sometimes pressed into backup medical duty, would watch Frances from a distance and mentally shake his head. Among others, two things amazed him about the field hospital routine: how Tiny Schwartz could whistle a song like "Stardust" while elbow-deep in a soldier's intestines. And how Frances Slanger, a Jewish nurse from just this side of poverty, had emerged as the best of the bunch.

She had, he had come to realize, an extraordinary sense of

purpose. Some of the enlisted men found Frances to be distant, even bossy. But she seemed to come alive in a medical tent—and not simply when looking into the eyes of Tiny Schwartz from across an operating stretcher. Frances saw hope in this maze of madness. Caring for the wounded drew on her die-hard belief that nursing was far more than the cold litany of procedures that Nurse Holland had taught back at Boston City Hospital. It was more than injecting a man with morphine to temporarily ease his physical pain, but injecting him with something as important: the desire to live. And here, in these mobile emergency rooms, she could work without some lemon-faced "snoopervisor" second-guessing her.

If Frances saw a need, say a patient unable to tip his head up to drink, she felt free to invent a better mousetrap, in one case an IV bottle with rubber tubing that allowed the patient to suck water. If a soldier wanted the bullet or a piece of the shrapnel that had hit him, she would make sure he got his souvenir. If she wanted to sing to some shell-shocked GI who had a vacant stare in his eyes, she sang.

And so as twilight turned to inky black on this late June night, the sky blessedly quiet because the cloud cover had grounded planes, Frances pulled up a wooden crate in the shock ward and took the mud-stained hand of the Tennessee boy. He desperately needed surgery but was still too weak. The summer rain played soft percussion on the tent. And in the dim light of the chamber of horrors, she quietly began to sing, "Let me call you sweetheart, I'm in love with you. . . ."

A hush instantly quieted the tent, as if a week-long storm had suddenly blown itself out. Soldiers, doctors, and other nurses paused. Eyes glistened as the soft song continued. "Let me hear you whisper that you love me, too / Keep the love light burning in your eyes so blue. . . ."

The soldier's eyebrows raised ever so slightly. His eyes

opened. He swallowed. At first, a touch of terror darted from his eyes as he struggled to orient himself. But, then, his expression calmed and his mouth opened ever so slowly.

"Hi . . . ya . . . babe," he said.

The wounded normally called the nurses "ma'am" or "lieu-tenant," but generally didn't talk much. The first thing they'd ask was how their buddy was, some guy who'd been hit in the same skirmish as they had. Complaints to nurses from soldiers were as rare as nights without ack-ack, a refreshing change from life in civilian hospitals back home.

Nurses would hide syringes when coming into a ward be-cause the soldier getting the shot didn't want his pals worrying about him. Occasionally, when a post-op nurse was called else-where, a soldier would sneak a cup of water for a buddy on the cot next to him. Such gestures touched the Forty-fifth's nurses. So, too, did the soldiers who would wake from a morphine-drugged state, their ears perhaps still ringing from the blast of a "screaming meemie," as GIs called the Germans' multiple-barreled rocket artillery. There above him was the face of a nurse. It was an epiphany of sorts, a man having fallen amid the stench of death, mud, and blood, and awakened to the smell of Woodhue perfume. Once, when a nurse reached across a GI to straighten his blanket, he kissed her arm. "I didn't know if I was dead or alive," he told her, "so I kissed you to see if you were an angel."

Part of the appeal, of course, was that the nurse was a woman; most soldiers hadn't seen one since leaving England weeks before, much less one riveting her attention directly on them. Even wearing no makeup except lipstick, and wearing fa-tigues or a simple brown-striped seersucker, wraparound dress, a nurse still had a certain diamond-in-the-rough appeal. She might not have been leggy actress Marlene Dietrich on a USO tour, but she was sanity in a world that had seemingly gone insane. She was a connection to home. And, above all, in this barbaric new world of kill-or-be-killed, she was the sweet manifestation of just the opposite: someone not trying to kill a man, but trying to keep him alive—and willing to share a stint in hell to do so.

"How . . . about . . . a . . . kiss?"

Frances Slanger loved those words, not for any romantic value but because of what they represented: the will to live. When Frances listened closely to war, she didn't hear distant gunfire, she heard heartbeats—and the aching silence when they stopped. Amid the horror of war, what inspired her most was the way a soldier who had arrived bloody and spent might resist the urge to die—the way he might, like a dying ember ignited by a wisp of wind, hang on to whatever life was still left in him.

The slight smile. The desire to ask for water or a cigarette, or even a kiss. To Frances, all whispered something achingly absent in her two weeks of war: hope.

She looked odd on the stretcher: a little French girl, lying doll-like in the middle of the canvas. She was placed in a post-op tent amid wounded men old enough to be her father. Men who had come to help set her free. Now this, the tragedy of liberation: She and her parents had returned to their home in a village and begun sifting through the rubble. A German booby trap exploded at their feet. Her parents died instantly. The little girl, about five years old, somehow survived the blast and the surgery, but her tiny body was splintered with shrapnel. She was unconscious, her face tinged a bluish green, most of her upper body wrapped in white bandages.

Michalove, making his daily rounds, closed the flap of the tent and walked away, pained by the sight of her. He wanted to cry, but then remembered who he was and where he was. He couldn't let his emotions get the best of him.

He was a softhearted man. A man touched when hearing

that his aunt and uncle back home had put his photo in the window of their Asheville clothing store along with one of their son, who was a marine in the South Pacific. A man for whom two weeks of war already seemed like two years.

He entered the mess tent—maybe a cup of joe would help him forget—and howdy'd Captain Shoham, his tent mate. When it came to food, Shoham and his Rebel underlings slopped on the tin plates whatever they had, from powdered eggs to canned vegetables to Spam. Shoham quickly learned that fresh meat of any kind appeased his customers—as long as he called it steak. His clientele was less enthralled with canned milk—"here comes the armored cow," a solider would say—and his coffee, which they likened to battery acid.

The only nurse Shoham had trouble with was Frances's tent mate, Elizabeth Powers, who was forever late turning orders in for her patients, even after Shoham threatened to go to Major Lord about it. But, generally, it was the enlisted men who complained most. "Hey," Shoham would remind them, "when you go home your wife is going to cook for you, your mom is going to cook for you, your girlfriend is going to cook for you. Here, I cook for you. Get used to it."

At times, the Second Platoon resorted to K-rations, a meal-in-a-box concoction that consisted of hardtack crackers, either cheese spread or potted meat, a fruit bar, an envelope of lemon crystals, and powdered coffee and sugar. Nearly everyone hated K-rations except for Michalove, who had made peace with the prepackaged meals. Like most soldiers, though, what he loved best was the farm-fresh eggs that the French would sometimes trade for American chocolate bars. Eggs were the ultimate taste of home.

While Michalove sipped his coffee, Shoham was trying to tear open a forty-pound box of packaged meat when he realized his tent mate was quieter than usual.

"You OK, Mike?" asked Shoham.

"Yeah, sure," said Michalove, sipping his coffee. But try as he might, he couldn't stop seeing the paratroopers hanging from the trees, swaying from their shrouds in the wind, helpless. And now this: the little orphaned French girl, fighting for life because of a war she'd had nothing to do with.

Michalove sipped his joe and tried to think about baseball on summer nights back home in Asheville.

IN THE MEDICAL TENTS, the wounded came and went like motel guests. The nurses had all seen the sick and the dead in the Stateside hospitals where they'd trained and worked, but this was different: not the eighty-year-old man whom time was tracking down or the chronically ill elderly woman, but strong, healthy soldiers—average age twenty-six. They were torn, bruised, and bloody, the dirt and shaveless days darkening their faces like death masks.

The enemy was real, and soldiers weren't the only ones in danger. In case a field hospital had to pack and leave because of approaching Germans, three people would need to stay behind with the wounded. It was a frightening proposition, all the more so given the thought of those left behind being Jewish; the Germans weren't as merciless as the Japanese when it came to prisoners, but were known to make exceptions for *Juden*.

Two days after the Second Platoon's arrival in Beuzeville au Plain, on the nineteenth, the worst June storm to hit the English Channel since the turn of the century ripped apart the artificial "Mulberry" harbor that was being built off Omaha Beach. The storm blew inland with a torrent of wind and rain, turning Normandy's roads and fields into mud that sucked boots like wet cement. For three days it hounded the Second Platoon's doctors and nurses, as if war alone wasn't challenging enough.

Field by field, surgery by surgery, the Battle of Normandy continued in a mind-numbing blur of blood and mud, the weather's only benefit being the temporary delay of the air war and blessed quiet. Finally, on June 27, American forces captured the port city of Cherbourg that was necessary before turning east toward Germany. What the American public saw of that event were triumphant wirephotos, including one of Sallylou Cummings smiling next to a severely wounded German POW, the First Platoon having gone to Cherbourg while the Second hung back. What the people back home didn't see was the hospital in Cherbourg that the Germans had vacated before American troops had swarmed in: a medical version of Dante's *Inferno*. Garbage cans literally teemed with severed arms and legs. There was no water to clean anything. The stench of gangrene and vomit and death assaulted the nostrils and sickened the stomach.

The next day, for the first time since leaving England, Sallylou went shopping. She bought a pair of cobalt blue earrings and a matching necklace.

By month's end, 27,000 American wounded had been evacuated to England. Eleven thousand were dead. And one thousand were nowhere to be found. For the Forty-fifth Field Hospital, the only silver lining in this cloud of grief was that in three weeks of intense combat, only one of their own—Berson, the dentist who'd been wounded the night the Forty-fifth had come ashore—was counted among those statistics. Still, the number of victims mounted.

"Blue 88s! Blue 88s!" yelled Frances, calling for tranquilizers so powerful they'd been jokingly renamed after the German artillery. In a frenzied pace that had become more norm than exception, Frances, other nurses, and medical technicians raced for bandages, fed soldiers bag after bag of blood and plasma, and took vitals. Though fewer than four percent of all patients admitted to a World War II field hospital died, in the early days in Normandy the Second Platoon was losing a far higher percentage: dozens of men a week—broken, maimed men who'd either lost the will to live or had no choice. Far more men than anyone had expected to lose.

Sgt. Charles Willen, a clerk in the Forty-fifth, once encountered a wounded soldier whom he'd trained with back in the States. The young man grabbed Willen's arm. "Don't let me die," he said. "Please don't let me die." But there was nothing Willen, or anyone else for that matter, could do. The soldier was too far gone.

The daily pile of bloody uniforms grew higher outside the tents. And the moans of soldiers became as much a part of the field hospital atmosphere as the nightly mantra of artillery fire and the incessant grind of the generator: *Mama, Mama* . . . Sometimes, such quiet pleas were stopped only by the gurgling of blood in the lungs, then death.

One soldier, an officer named Lieutenant Flowers, came to the Second Platoon's tent needing to have both legs amputated. His face writhed in agony, which turned to anger a few days later when a couple of brass hats dropped by the post-op tent to pin a Purple Heart on the now-legless man. "What am I good for when I get home?" he muttered to Shoham.

Later, another GI, hardly more than a boy, needed to have a leg removed. Nurse Betty Belanger learned that he'd lied about his age because he was so anxious to enlist. Frantically, doctors tried to anesthetize him for surgery but nothing would work. Fear held him hostage. Finally, Betty did the only thing she could think of: leaned over and cradled him in her arms.

When first arriving in Normandy, she had begun a journal. But she soon stopped. It was too painful remembering days like this one. And the one before it. And the one that would follow.

• • •

JOHN BONZER, his surgical mask wicked with sweat, looked up from the abdominal spaghetti—some soldier who'd gotten married the week before he'd left for Europe but whose young wife was on the verge of becoming a widow.

"They're all just kids," he muttered to nobody in particular. "Just *kids*, damn it."

Two weeks of nearly nonstop surgery had left Bonzer—at twenty-five, nearly a kid himself—emotionally spent as he assisted Third Auxiliary surgeons. But for all the tangled emotions that doctors and nurses felt, they could steel themselves against such emotions because of the necessity to perform. The nonmedical soldiers such as Michalove didn't have such protection; they had time to observe, ponder, plot. Some in the Forty-fifth found comfort in prayer, others in black humor, others in 180-proof grain alcohol mixed with grapefruit juice, a concoction so powerful—"screech," they called it—and so much in demand among the enlisted men that the Forty-fifth's officers began coloring it blue to discourage its use.

Michalove was having difficulty finding comfort anywhere. While making his rounds, he had seen far too many nurses pull blankets over the faces of lifeless GIs. He was still haunted by the sight of the dangling paratroopers. And, moments before, Shoham had broken the news to him.

"Mike, the little girl . . . We lost her."

Later, Michalove walked to the edge of camp, near a hedgerow, a man awash in a blend of anger and despair. Somewhere in the cloudy distance, a wounded horse neighed. Slowly, as if by some force other than his own, Michalove raised the back of a clenched fist to his mouth. Not too long ago he had been wrapped in the innocence of hawking hot dogs at baseball games. Now this: The blood. The hopelessness. It was all too much for—

Something moved behind him. Michalove slowly turned. There stood Frances Slanger, her too-large helmet, as usual, tilted back.

"Close your eyes, Captain," said Frances, reaching for something in her field jacket pocket.

"For you," she said, and placed it in the palm of his hand. It was a farm-fresh egg, still warm. Michalove took the gift, stared at it as if were made of gold, and looked up at Frances.

He began to cry.

CHAPTER 8

He has achieved success who has lived well, laughed often and loved much . . . who has filled his niche and accomplished his task; who has left the world better than he found it, whether by an improved poppy, a perfect poem, or a rescued soul. . . .

—MRS. A. J. STANLEY,
FOUND IN FRANCES SLANGER'S CHAPBOOK

Like most wounded soldiers, he'd arrived with eyes filled with fear. Frances had been beside him much of the night. She dabbed his forehead with a damp rag, gave him sips of water, and asked questions about his hometown. Shoham joked with Frances that it was no good trying to talk books and authors with these guys. "Talk to them about baseball. Talk to them about Boston's Bobby Doerr and Fenway Park." Frances had rolled her eyes in response.

Like most soldiers, this one didn't talk much, though more than most, particularly considering the German machine gun had not only shredded his colon, but had also chipped off part of his chin. His eyes, though, seemed to have brightened, which did the same for her. She liked him. Ever since Lødz, Frances had always liked an underdog.

Post-op was its usual chaotic self. Frances moved from cot to cot, giving shots, changing dressings, and soothing fears in what, by now, had become a routine weighted in fatigue. As her twelve-hour night shift neared its 8 A.M. end, her face was smudged with a weariness that she willed herself to hide. Still, when finding time, she checked back with the soldier, talking to him of life after all this. She whispered encouragement, prayed her prayers, and, finally, pulled up a crate and held the man's hand, her encouragement feeding off his encouragement. "I shall appear fearless in the presence of danger," said a portion of the "Pledge of the Army Nurse," "and quiet the fears of others to the best of my ability."

Suddenly, though, the soldier's eyes grew hollow. Frances tensed. *No, this can't happen. Hang on, soldier, hang on.* She dug deep for whatever resolve she had, some rooftop poem she'd written about never giving up, some prayer she'd first prayed when the bloody German soldiers had taken over Łódz. *Hang on. You're going home, remember? You're somebody's son.*

His hand squeezed her hand hard, then went limp. His eyes stared at something beyond her. She checked his pulse. The soldier was dead. Just like that. Gone. For Frances, it was the harshest of lessons: the realization that hopes and prayers and talk of home were sometimes no match for shrapnel and bullets and rifle butts used to bludgeon human flesh. She slowly walked backward, not wanting to believe it. She pursed her lips together, wanting to cry. Instead, she did what she had been doing since she was a little girl: She blamed herself.

It had always been this way for Frances. Years before, in Boston, she'd captured her never-good-enough lament in a poem she wrote called "End of the Nurse's Day":

Seven o'clock and the nurse
Was done for another day
She heaved a tired sigh
And put the charts away.

Then sat for a moment and bowed her head,
Over the little white desk.
I wonder, said she to herself,
Am I really doing my best?
Perhaps I could have begun the day
With a brighter, cheerier smile.
And answered the bells with "Right away"
Instead of, "After a while."
And I might have listened with sweeter grace
To the tale of Six's woes.
She may be suffering more, perhaps
More than anyone knows.
And I might have refrained from the
Halfway frown,
Although I was busy then,
When that frail little girl with sad blue eyes
Kept ringing again and again.
And I might have spoken a kinder word,
To the heart of that restless boy
And stopped a moment to help him find
The missing part to his toy.
Or perhaps the patient in 18A
Just needed a gentler touch,
There are a lot of things I might have done,
And it wouldn't have taken much.
She sighed again then brushed a tear,
And whispered praying low,
My God, how can you accept this day,
When it has been lacking so?
And God looked down, he heard that sigh
And saw that shining tear,
Then sent his angel messenger
To whisper in her ear.

You could have done better today
But, oh, the omnipotent one
Seeing your faults does not forget
The beautiful things you have done.
He knows, little nurse, that you love your work
In this house of pain and sorrow
So forgives the lack of today,
For you will do better tomorrow.
The nurse looked up with a grateful smile,
Tomorrow I'll make it right
Then added a note in her order book:
"Be good to them tonight."

In a field hospital, the ultimate "house of pain and sorrow," Frances was learning that the stakes were far higher than at Boston City Hospital, and offered little time for grief. Around her, the never-ending challenge of saving lives continued. Soldiers moaned softly. Doctors and their surgical assistants cut, clipped, and clamped with less emotion than if they were working on an assembly line. Nurses flitted from patient to patient. Nobody but Frances even noticed that another soldier had died. She took one last look at the young man whose death would break hearts when word reached home, then pulled the army blanket over his face. In moments, two privates whisked the dead man away. One of his buddies needed the cot.

IN EARLY JULY, the Second Platoon's convoy was slowly snaking its way through the French countryside, near a village named Orglandes, when it came upon what looked to be a deserted farm. A group of enlisted men, rifles at the ready, went from room to room, kicking in doors. Finding nobody, they ventured outside the house. A lone dead German soldier lay draped over a fence; other bodies were scattered in a field. A slight noise rustled from behind a barn. One of the enlisted men, his back to the side of the stone-block structure, slid to an outside corner. A group of doctors and nurses, including Frances, watched from a distance. So did three German POWs whom the Second was shepherding until the enemy soldiers could be turned over to the military police.

The American soldier raised his rifle, the muzzle pointed skyward. His eyes darted right and left. He pivoted around at the corner, aimed his weapon, then felt the adrenaline drain from his body. He laughed nervously, then again.

"Ducks," he called back. "We got ourselves ducks!"

By now, Captain Shoham's Rebels had become adroit at one-handing any meat-flanked bird within reach. In moments, nine ducks were dead and ready for gutting. Not far away, amid a cluster of the seventy-plus people in the platoon, came a complementary find: a barrel of grain alcohol. After a nurse's quick consultation with Major Lord, an enlisted man whistled to get everyone's attention and one of the nurses announced it on the spot.

"A party!" she said. "Offered by the Second Platoon nurses to the entire outfit, at 1800. Dress: Casual. The menu: Du—"

"Steak!" interrupted Shoham, a line that triggered hoots and hollers, everyone knowing by now that their chief cook called any meat he had, including Spam, "steak." And so the Second Platoon, only too happy to forget what their lives had become, partied as darkness descended, the Normandy night filled with the smell of sizzling meat. At one point, the three German POWs, who'd been helping the cooks with cleanup, asked permission to bury the German soldier draped over the fence. They were allowed to do so, digging a grave amid an apple orchard and burying their comrade, decorating his resting spot with a belt of fifty-caliber American machine-gun ammunition.

Giving such freedom to POWs wasn't uncommon; the prisoners were given a number of jobs around camp and, besides, bullets without guns were no threat to anyone.

In a field near the quiet ceremony, the Second Platoon drank, smoked, and danced to records played on a phonograph—five songs, repeating themselves over and over. A couple of fights between well-potted enlisted men broke out and were quickly doused. Across the way, Tiny Schwartz towered above the throng with uncharacteristic brashness, conducting the phonograph "band" with a tree twig. Others in the Forty-fifth were far more likely to see him huddling with some weary-of-war pal—"the father confessor," as Shoham called him. But every now and then, Schwartz, like Slanger, could be like a little kid, with a smile that didn't end.

Frances watched him from afar, smiling slightly. The five songs repeated until, her mind softened by the alcohol, she'd almost felt as if she were back in North Carolina, where she'd first met the man whom everyone called "Tiny" but she thought of as "Isadore," where she'd met most of these compatriots who were now part of this traveling medical circus. And where, for the first time in her life, she actually felt she belonged.

AT FORT BRAGG, the white, two-story barracks on this cold morning stretched on seemingly forever, as stark and neatly lined up as frosted dogwoods at a tree nursery. It was early February 1944. A skiff of overnight snow had starched the branches of loblolly pines and the sandy soil of the camp, which stretched seventy-four square miles across the eastern hills of North Carolina.

A photographer stood on a trunk and, using a megaphone, tried yelling instructions to more than two hundred uniformed men and women who were reluctantly positioning themselves on four rows of bleachers. It was picture day for the U.S. Army's Forty-fifth Field Hospital Unit, which would soon be leaving for Europe.

Nearby, soldiers, singing a cadence to keep time, marched down dirt roads flanked by the cookie-cutter barracks—not to be confused with the cookie-cutter barracks for the "colored troops," which were in a separate location on the post. Trucks and jeeps rumbled by, leaving behind a hint of reddish dust and the lingering smell of diesel.

As the photographer begged for the members of the Forty-fifth to squeeze in, the unit froze in a pose of seriousness that looked to be part military obedience and part children-forced-to-eat-spinach. More than a few among the Forty-fifth were nursing hangovers from what had become known as "priming the pump" in Fayetteville, a town eleven miles away. There, the Town Pump bar welcomed slews of military personnel—and later "unwelcomed" a good many in the wakes of brawls. Oftentimes, paratroopers from the 82nd and 101st Airborne Divisions wound up pitted against ground troops because of exaggerated egos among the jumpers, latent jealousy among the others, or a combination of the two. At times, guys from the 101st took on guys from the 82nd, paratroopers took on glider troops, or whites sparred with blacks. Given such tinderbox potential, nurses found themselves more than welcome at the Town Pump. They drew business, bought drinks, and didn't fight. What more could a bar owner ask for?

For the photo, the 208 men of the Forty-fifth wore tan chinos, dark olive-drab blouses, and beige ties. The eighteen women, all nurses, wore their "Class A" dress uniforms: brownish green skirts, blouses, shirts, and ties. Everybody wore gloves and garrison caps.

Except for a Sgt. "Utah" Jackson, an Indian from Oklahoma,

BOB WELCH

and a few Hispanics, including Pvt. Vincente Rivas of New Mexico, everyone in the Forty-fifth was white; "Negroes," by law, were segregated from white units. For a country fighting the bigotry of Hitler, the hypocrisy seemed achingly obvious to some. During the early forties, however, the government wouldn't budge on segregation, even after lynchings, riots, and constant pressure from the National Association for the Advancement of Colored People.

The uniformity among the Forty-fifth accentuated the few visual oddities in the group, one of which was a mountain of a man in the front row, Isadore Schwartz, a six-foot-three, 250-pound physician from Quincy, Massachusetts. His nickname had long been "Itzie," but at Fort Bragg he'd quickly been dubbed "Tiny."

As the photographer tripped the shutter for a shot, Schwartz stood tall with a sheepish grin on his face and eyes almost totally closed, a look that begged the question: Who is this guy and what's he doing here? He seemed an odd fit for the military and, given his size, odder still for the medical profession. But Schwartz was deceptively sharp and dependable. He had not only graduated magna cum laude from Tufts University in Boston, but had managed to ace his medical exams even though he'd played trumpet at a senior prom in Providence, Rhode Island, partied most of the night, and arrived at the test site still wearing his tux. When he arrived at Fort Bragg, he was twenty-six years old and had been married six years.

A row back and fifteen feet to his left stood the shortest person in the unit, Frances Slanger. At five-foot-one, she was dwarfed by fellow nurses, not to mention doctors and enlisted men. But she stood tall. She looked slightly away from the camera, not straight at it as others did, as if either self-conscious or her mind was somewhere else. Perhaps both.

Schwartz and Slanger, respectively, were the tallest and

146

shortest members of the entire Forty-fifth, ironic since they were so similar in other ways. Above all, both lived in unrelenting pursuit of goodness, even if it meant bucking the status quo to achieve it. In fact, that's why both were standing on these bleachers in the first place—because, in pursuit of an ideal, they'd dared to question military decisions they believed to be wrong.

Frances had argued that she belonged overseas; the army, ultimately, agreed. Schwartz's pathway to the Forty-fifth was different. Originally, he'd been ticketed for Stateside service because of a bad back and bad feet. The latter, he believed, was the result of Mr. Kutz, the Schwartz family's shoe peddler; refusing to believe Isadore could have size 13 shoes, he continually gave the boy size 10.

But Schwartz's military status changed at Fort Bragg. As a Jew, Schwartz had known prejudice. He'd initially been blocked from enrolling at Tufts because of a quota system limiting the number of Jewish applicants. He'd heard the anti-Semitic radio ramblings of Father Charles Coughlin, whose Sunday afternoon messages were a favorite among many of Boston's Irish-Catholic families. He'd grown up in the greater Boston area, where youth gangs vandalized Jewish cemeteries, synagogues were defaced with swastikas, and anti-Semitic literature was widely distributed, some during World War II deriding Jews for not carrying their weight in battle. Now, he'd become part of a U.S. military system that was openly racist, particularly in the South, and it boiled a dormant rage within.

Training programs were segregated. Blacks were rarely given more than menial jobs. In the early years of the war, black nurses treated only black patients. In a letter to *Yank* magazine, a black soldier described how a Texas railroad depot had made black GIs go around back to the kitchen for sandwiches and coffee and, meanwhile, happily served two dozen German POWs out front. At Fort Bragg, a fight had broken out between blacks and whites on the way into Fayetteville. In the aftermath, hundreds of black soldiers—most nowhere near the incident—were herded into the base stockade, where many were beaten by guards.

Schwartz was not only a Jew, but an Orthodox Jew, a letter-of-the-law man who spoke his mind. When he arrived at Fort Bragg and found "White" and "Colored" signs for toilet facilities in the hospital ward he was to oversee, he immediately ordered them taken down. When Schwartz's superior found out, the commanding officer was livid. Schwartz was punished for his insubordination with a new assignment: overseas duty. There, he would befriend a nurse named Frances Slanger, whose life would forever be intertwined with his.

THE FORT BRAGG barracks were a study in visual sameness: more than 300 identical buildings each housing sixty-three people all lined up, with equal space between them, like so many cookies on a sheet. Functionality, not ambience, was the goal here. Only at the insistence of First Lady Eleanor Roosevelt, after a tour of the fort, had such quarters even been slapped with a coat of paint.

Inside one such barrack, the *click-click-click* of typewriter keys and the *zip-ding* of a carriage return added an odd touch to a February evening in 1944. Frances Slanger was at it again. "Tell me when you complete your first best seller," Margaret Morrison, a Forty-fifth nurse from Nova Scotia, told her.

Frances smiled and kept typing.

The Forty-fifth's nurses spent part of their time at Fort Bragg bivouacked in the North Carolina woods, beneath pine trees. But much of their time at Bragg was spent in barracks that were boringly similar, each soldier or nurse having a bed and footlocker at the foot of that bed, shoes underneath, uniforms grouped on a nearby wall rack.

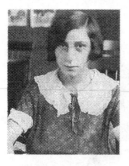

At twelve, Frances, here in a photo at Abraham Lincoln School, lived the life of a "go-between." It was a common plight for immigrant children: running errands for their foreign-speaking parents because the children learned English so much faster. Even as an adult, Frances would find herself something of a go-between, becoming the family's major financial support. *(Sidman family collection)*

Slanger, here at age seventeen or eighteen in 1931, cherished her time at Cape Cod. She once wrote in a poem: "How I wish I were now in Cape Cod / Where the tree tops gently seem to nod / Where the . . . breezes softly blow / Where the larkspur and snapdragon grow . . ." *(Sidman family collection)*

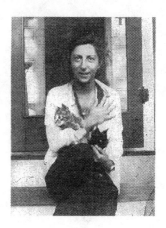

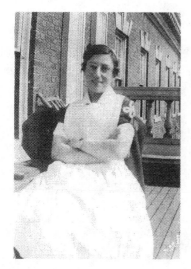

Despite some supervisors who said she wasn't nursing material, Frances earned her credentials at Boston City Hospital, graduating in 1937. Even as a young girl she had wanted to be a nurse. "I want to serve [those] who are less fortunate than I," she wrote. "I have always loved to comfort those who were sick." *(Sidman family collection)*

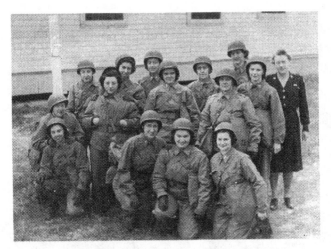

At Fort Bragg, North Carolina, shortly before the 45th Field Hospital shipped out to England, the nurses posed in front of one of the cookie-cutter barracks. Frances is fourth from the left, hands in pocket. Behind her, with her hands on Frances's shoulders, is a tent mate, Christine Cox. To the far right: Capt. Elizabeth Hay. *(Courtesy of the Boston Public Library, Print Department)*

During training, beneath the pine trees of Fort Bragg, in February 1944, Frances Slanger (standing, far right) and nurses from the 45th Field Hospital take a break. As was often the case, Frances found herself on the fringe of a group, sometimes by choice, sometimes not. *(John Bonzer collection)*

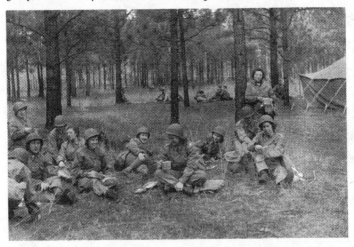

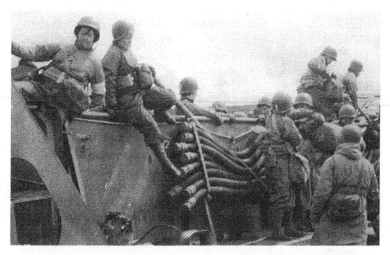

Some of the 45th Field Hospital's eighteen nurses prepare to leave their landing craft to go ashore at the Uncle Red sector of Utah Beach on June 10, 1944. The 45th's eighteen women, along with those from the 128th Evacuation Hospital, were the first American nurses to step foot in France during WWII. *(Dottie Richter Lewis collection)*

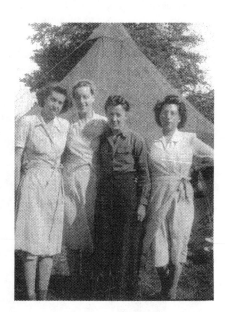

Frances (far right) with her tent mates (left to right) Christine Cox, Elizabeth Powers, and Margaret Bowler. The Massachusetts nurses met at basic training at Fort Devens, near Boston, and were together in the very end, huddled in a tent during a surprise German attack. *(From the Frances Slanger Collection in the Howard Gotlieb Archival Research Center at Boston University)*

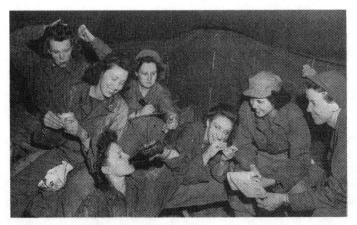

Contrived scenes such as this, shot by an Army photographer long before the 45th left the states for England, created an image of levity among nurses that proved to be the exception, not the rule, in war. Nurses worked twelve-hour shifts and were usually too tired to do anything else but sleep when not on duty. *(U.S. Army)*

Nurses tend to "patients" in a stateside setup for an Army photographer. Once in France, such calm, antiseptic scenes gave way to considerably more grit and chaos. As in the photo, soldiers on cots were lined on each side of the tent's outer edges, alternating directions so one man wouldn't be as apt to spread germs to another. *(U.S. Army)*

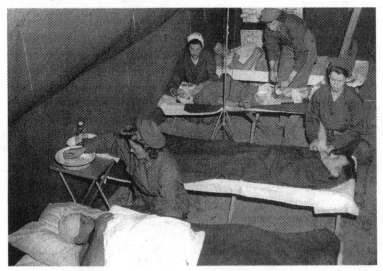

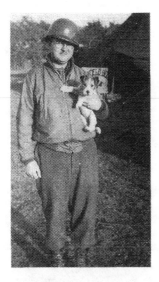

Shortly before a surprise German attack, Major Herman Lord strolled the camp with Penny, the wire-haired terrier that the Second Platoon had picked up after the liberation of Paris. Lord, married and from Detroit, leaned to the frumpy side, but was respected as a dependable leader and was—said one staff sergeant—"one swell surgeon." *(John Bonzer collection.)*

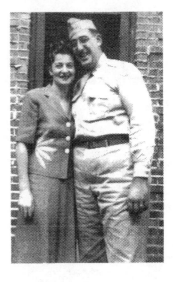

Isadore "Tiny" Schwartz with his wife, Ruth Sherman, whom he'd married before the war. From afar, some wondered if Schwartz and Frances Slanger weren't more than just friends, but those who knew the two best thought otherwise: kindred spirits, yes; lovers, no. *(Edward Schwartz collection)*

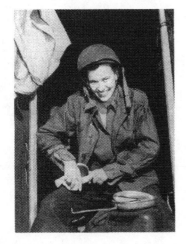

After the war, *The Saturday Evening Post* chose Sallylou Cummings to feature in a major spread on nurses. Here, at the request of the *Post* photographer, she models the typical nursing outfit she wore when she was with the 45th Field Hospital in Europe. *(Reprinted with permission of* The Saturday Evening Post, © 1948 [Renewed], BFL&MS, Inc. Indianapolis)*

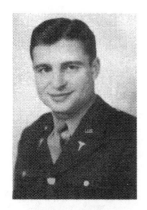

Dr. John Bonzer fell in love with Frances Slanger's polar opposite, Sallylou Cummings, in England while the 45th Field Hospital was waiting for the D Day Invasion to begin. But once in France, the two wound up in separate platoons. Bonzer was part of the Second Platoon, which included Frances, a woman whom Bonzer found took nursing—and life—more seriously than most, even if she did call him "Johnny." *(John Bonzer collection)*

Capt. Joseph Shoham, a dentist and cook in the 45th's 2nd Platoon, may have understood Frances Slanger better than anyone. "You go through your life thinking: 'What could I have done?' " he says. "She *did* it. She left the world better than she found it." *(John Bonzer collection)*

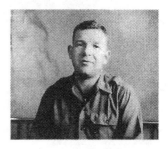

Two weeks after Frances Slanger's editorial was published in *Stars and Stripes*, the military newspaper broke the news of her death. Both articles triggered scores of poignant letters from GIs in France, Belgium, Luxembourg, and Germany.

Wrote one G.I., Pvt. Jack Hoss: "Gallant heroines and heroes always die a gallant death." *(Stars and Stripes)*

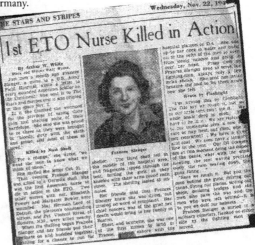

Frances Slanger is a great woman. We say is — because her memory in our minds will linger steadfastly long after the final gun is fired in this war. Why ??? Because Frances Slanger pointed out the only genuine rule for peace on earth. Human love and understanding.

Slanger's letter to *Stars and Stripes* and subsequent death triggered hundreds of letters from American soldiers across Europe, including this one from Sgt. George W. Fritton, an air gunner with the Army Air Force's 647th Bomb Squad, 410 Bomb Group. Eight other airmen signed the letter. *(National Archives)*

In November 1947, more than two years after the war had ended, Frances's body was returned to America. In Boston, hundreds came to pay their respects, but only one doctor from the 45th Field Hospital: Isadore Schwartz. Elizabeth Powers, wounded in the same blast that had killed her tent mate, knelt at the casket. "Hello, soldier," she whispered. *(Boston Public Library)*

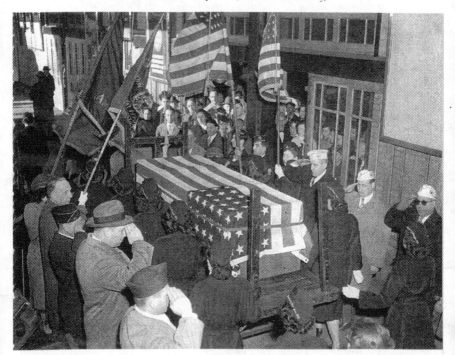

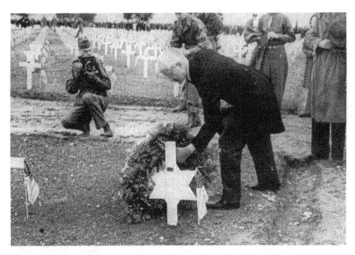

Charles Sawyer, the U.S. ambassador to Belgium, places a wreath on the marker of Frances Slanger's grave at Henri-Chapelle Cemetery in Belgium during a Memorial Day commemoration on May 30, 1945. Sawyer gave a speech that referred to President Franklin D. Roosevelt, but spent far more time talking about Slanger. "We thank you for the things you have said about the GIs," said Sawyer, as if he were talking to Frances herself. "They are better said by you than by any other. If there is in heaven and in our hearts a special shrine for those who have given the most and the best, it is held sacred for the American nurse." Gen. Dwight Eisenhower was among those in the audience. *(U.S. Army, from the Frances Slanger Collection in the Howard Gotlieb Archival Research Center at Boston University)*

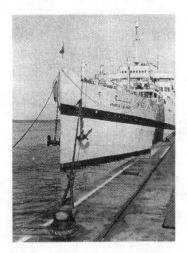

After its maiden voyage from New York, the *Frances Y. Slanger* hospital ship stopped in Southampton, England, in July 1945 after picking up wounded soldiers in Cherbourg, France. The *Slanger* was the largest and fastest ship in the hospital fleet. *(John Bonzer collection)*

On their rare evenings off, most of the Forty-fifth's nurses headed for Fayetteville, a few dozen tobacco and cotton fields away. After the boredom of Bragg, the nurses clutched their bus-line scrip as if they were tickets to heaven. The odds alone were intriguing: about one hundred men for every woman. One night, Monty reluctantly agreed to go dancing with a smart-aleck lieutenant named Edward Bowen, the administrator of the field hospital's First Platoon. She was dreading the date. But the two danced away the evening and by morning they were in love.

Frances declined trips to Fayetteville. Those who knew her shrugged it off as simply "Frances being Frances"—she's just *reserved*, they'd say—but others took it as an outright snub. Frances wasn't everybody's cup of joe. Some, particularly among the enlisted men who didn't know her well, found her icy. All business, no fun. The kind of girl who had to have knock-knock jokes explained to her. And given her plain-Jane looks, not exactly anyone's dream date.

"Screw her," an enlisted man once muttered to Sgt. Charles Willen, a twenty-two-year-old clerk from Delaware, after Frances had finger-wagged the guy for not taking his job more seriously.

If Frances seemed cold to the enlisted men, it was, in part, because they were, beyond hospital orderlies, the first group of people she'd had authority over. Her entire life, Frances had been told what to do. Now, as an army lieutenant, she had people who answered to her—or at least were supposed to. Lieutenants answered to captains. Doctors were captains or higher in rank; the commanding officer of the Second Platoon, for example, was Herman Lord, a major. But privates, the enlisted men, answered to lieutenants. If a nurse knew the field hospital was running low on, say, blankets, she could order a private to do something about it. It was hard enough for some men to take orders from a woman, harder still from a five-foot-one woman, and, in this case, a *Jewish* woman.

What's more, she had little patience with those who lacked compassion for others. Her patriotism was rooted deep; MacArthur's "I will return" promise, she'd once written, had "singed itself into my soul." If she saw the military as a serious mission, a means-to-an-end way of trying to stop the human suffering going on in the world, many of the enlisted men saw it as a whopping pain in the butt. And while a few nurses won over enlisted men in bars or beds, Frances wasn't among them.

By now, she had made four stops on this Army Nurse Corps tour: Fort Devens in Massachusetts, Fort Rucker in Alabama, Camp Gordon in Georgia, and Fort Bragg in North Carolina. Most nurses and doctors saw her as a loner but not necessarily unfriendly. Evelyn Moore, who had roomed with Frances at Devens, had told her she was one of the "truest friends" she'd ever found. At Camp Gordon, Pvt. Ben Schwartz had told her how proud he was of the friendship they'd forged. Still, being part of a group had never been easy for Frances; around people, her insecurities increased. At some point in her past, someone— a man?—had taken advantage of her in a way that wounded her deeply, or so her poetry suggests: "You are the flame, I am the moth/You lure me on, and you care not."

Meanwhile, her lower-class upbringing wasn't point-scoring potential at any social gathering. *And I'd like to introduce you to Frances Slanger, whose family has never owned property even the size of a postage stamp, much less a car. She's a fruit peddler's daughter!* In some ways, being part of any kind of relationship was difficult for her. Beyond that, Frances simply liked spending time alone. She was, after all, a writer. *Goodness, Millay hadn't won her Pulitzer without holing herself up now and then by herself; this is what writers do.* Which is why Frances, while most of the Forty-fifth did their best to implode the once-sleepy town of Fayetteville, stayed behind.

At Fort Devens, Capt. Bertha Grady, after reading some of Frances's poetry, not only approved of her writing but challenged her to get some of it published. At first, Frances had shaken her head no; she'd never been published beyond some short stories and poetry in her high school literary magazine and a few one-liners in the *Boston Herald*. But as Grady persisted, Frances reluctantly took that challenge. She wrote a piece on the rigors of training, then sent it to the *Boston Traveler* newspaper. The paper published the piece, an editor saying he'd never seen the written perspective of an army nurse before. The article was also printed in the *American Journal of Nursing* and in the *Fort Devens Digest*. In one part, Frances described an obstacle course.

> Not being athletically inclined, I was scared to death when I saw the obstacles. No telling what would happen here. There were three hurdles of different heights which we had to jump or climb over, an upright wall of logs we had to scale; a shallow ditch which we had to cross by swinging over with a rope (something that Tarzan does in the movies, you know); and, finally, a series of bars suspended over another shallow ditch.
>
> When it was my turn to jump the hurdles, about six of us went together. It made it a little easier to see the others struggle too. I jumped the first hurdle. I climbed over the second, but the third one got me. I tried to cheat and go under it but the lynx-eyed lieutenant saw me and said, "Ah, ah, not nice . . . over not under." I tried going around it. No good. He saw me again. I tried throwing one leg over but the other one remained fixed to the ground. Then I tried throwing my whole weight over it, but the law of gravity was against me.
>
> Finally, with a gentle shove from the lieutenant

(which almost landed me on my head) I was over! I felt quite proud.

For someone whose lack of self-esteem had anchored her to self-perceived failure, Frances found six months at four training camps freeing. She overcame hurdles she thought insurmountable. She got published. And she got praised. "You'll make it if you are as good a writer as you are a nurse," Margaret Morrison told her. The *American Journal of Nursing* contacted Captain Grady about getting more stories from Frances. "Lt. Slanger writes so entertainingly," wrote Nell V. Beeby, the magazine's assistant editor.

For someone whose lack of independence had prevented her from seeing just how high she could fly, the army allowed Frances the chance to test herself. "We all feel quite ready and even anxious to go anywhere and do what is expected of us to the greatest of our ability," she'd written in the final part of her published story on basic training. "We are proud to be members of the United States Army." But editors had deleted a clause from the last line of her original version, which ended: "We are glad to have severed those ties that held us down and are proud to be members of the United States Army." It was a telling phrase— "glad to have severed those ties that held us down"—and only confirmed Frances's new sense of freedom.

Finally, for someone whose lack of adventure had limited the latitude of her writing, the army gave Frances a chance to meet new people, see new places, and face new experiences. Though she never imagined herself marching in a War Bonds parade in Dothan, Alabama, or battling cockroaches while taking temperatures at a Fort Rucker, Alabama, hospital, the experiences were at least something different from the routine at Boston City. Though they were as basic as white bread, she found the quarters at Camp Gordon in Georgia "lovely"—the nurses "grand." "We have been accepted, not only as fellow nurses, but like friends of long standing," she wrote. "In a sense, we almost hate to leave these girls. There are many pleasant memories we are taking with us."

When it was time to head for Fort Bragg, her fellow nurses chose Frances to write a good-bye piece for the *Camp Gordon Cadence*. Earlier, she had written about being on night patrol, and about Captain Grady of her Devens days. In the latter poem, Frances even allowed her lighter side to come out and play, a rarity for her:

> I don't know what I'm rooting for
> Down here they're fighting the Civil War
> and now at last we're doing nights
> helping patients and scratching bites. . . .

The much-longer poem, written while on night duty, was a tribute to Grady, who was—in Frances's eyes—both a "soldier and a lady." " . . . She stands so straight and salutes so smart / This business is rooted deep in her heart. . . ."

And so, too, was this business beginning to root itself deep in Frances's heart—as were her peers. Doctors and nurses and other officers kidded her about her *Bawston* accent, her bunk area being obsessively neat, and her shrill voice, the audio equivalent of coffee so strong you could not only taste, but *feel*, the grounds. She responded by occasionally breaking into falsetto.

In December 1943, two months before leaving for Europe, Frances sent homemade Christmas cards to friends back in Boston featuring a front-door wreath powdered with snow. A few weeks later she sent her mother a certificate confirming her status as part of the U.S. Army Nurse Corps. It included a photo of herself, surrounded by separate photographs of President

Franklin Roosevelt, Chief of Staff General George C. Marshall, Secretary of War Henry Stimson and her hero, Gen. Douglas MacArthur, commanding general of Allied Forces in the Southwest Pacific.

"To a swell little mother," she wrote on the photograph. "Love, Frances."

THE FORTY-FIFTH left for England in the early morning darkness of February 27, 1944, a Sunday. While New Yorkers slept beneath a blanket of fresh snow, tugs eased a 492-foot ship out of her slip at the New York Port of Embarkation and pointed her bow east in the oil-black waters of the Hudson River. Her name, appropriate enough given the nurses on board, was the USS *Florence Nightingale.* A few snowflakes twirled harmlessly in the lights of the ship. As the vessel glided, ghostlike, past Ellis Island in the darkness, its starboard wake slapped against the rock seawall in splashes of irony: Frances Slanger, the little girl once nearly blocked from entering this country, was now heading off to help defend it.

As Frances settled in on a bunk deep in the guts of the ship, it had been six months since she'd left home for Fort Devens. She'd met dozens of new people, some of whom left their farewells in an autograph book that she now read by flashlight while lying on her bunk.

"We never did double-date but we will someday in Brooklyn, OK?" wrote Roslyn L. Tauber of New York.

"Frances, dear," wrote Louis A. Patterson of Los Angeles, "I hope we will be friends long after the war is forgotten."

Frances C. Ryer, a nurse from Canada, thought it appropriate to leave her poet friend a poem:

The days of skipping rope, now are past
The voice of high opera gone at last

The clang of the typewriter heard no more
It's not like home since you closed our door.

The *Florence Nightingale* churned into the darkness beyond. Frances turned off her flashlight and soon fell asleep to the thrum of the engines, each revolution of the single propeller moving her farther away from home—and closer to where she knew she must be.

CHAPTER 9

I am footsore and very weary,
But I travel to meet a friend,
The way is so long and dreary,
But I know that it soon must end.
He is traveling fast like the whirlwind.
And though I creep slowly on,
He is coming ever nearer,
And the journey is almost done.

—ANONYMOUS,
FOUND IN FRANCES SLANGER'S CHAPBOOK

The morning sun hadn't soaked into the tent for more than an hour but already Frances Slanger's canvas home was turning warm. The sky was blue. Bees and flies—nature's buzz bombs—began their annoying morning sorties. The summer heat sharpened the musty smell of canvas and moldy boots, one reminder to Frances that this wasn't Roxbury. The other reminder was that her body was one solid ache.

So where was this place that they'd arrived at the previous day? And what day of the week was it? And even if she knew the answers to both questions, what did it really matter? Nearly a month into the Battle of Normandy, life at war had become life

without context. As the Forty-fifth Field Hospital's three platoons leapfrogged across France, the nurses had no idea what
was happening ahead of or behind them, except for what they
might hear through mess tent scuttlebutt. Frances and the others never saw the wounded before they arrived nor after they'd
left. The nurses moved when told, from places they didn't know
to new places they didn't know. And, as summer deepened, the
pattern repeated itself with a numbing sameness.

Frances slapped a mosquito on her arm. By now, some of
the nurses were well pocked by the insects that infested
hedgerows. She dug through her musette bag for toothpaste and
brush, a laughable task given how much she'd brought and how
little she actually needed. No wonder Shoham complained that
lifting nurses' gear had thrown out his back: besides gobs of
clothes she never wore, Frances carried a dog-eared notebook,
two address books, a box of crayons, a flashlight, a camera, two
fountain pens, three erasers, two family photographs, twenty-
two handkerchiefs, a Star of David emblem, one official Boston
Police pass, and a Boston City Hospital ring. The nurses weren't
allowed to wear jewelry, though lipstick was encouraged. It
raised the men's morale, higher-ups believed.

Locked into a routine that, by now, required little thought,
Frances poured water from a French pitcher that she and her tent
mates had picked up somewhere along the way—*les someplace* or
some such name she couldn't pronounce—and washed her face.
She brushed her teeth, hung her towel on one of the nails pro-
truding from the main tent pole, opened the tent flap, and spit.

From the French pitcher, she poured some water into her
overturned helmet to wash her face. The practice had begun in
Bristol, England, where the nurses had been billeted in a place
called Tortworth Castle, whose turrets and stone regality were
framed with rhododendrons and shrubs. A most unlikely place
for army personnel, it was there that some in the Forty-fifth had

met war correspondent Ernie Pyle, who was visiting a pal from the 128th Evac. And there that the nurses realized they were without working baths or showers. That meant taking sponge baths out of their helmets, a crude, if effective way, of getting clean. "Your seat, your feet, and under your arms," went the protocol.

The first time a handful of nurses tried taking a bath out of their helmets, Betty Belanger laughed at this experiment in primitive cleansing. "Brrrrr," she said, after tipping a helmet of cold water down her back. "Where I'm from, we used to call these 'Jewish baths.'" Her words had barely left her mouth when she realized who else was in the room: Frances, across from her in the dimly lit circle. Betty was mortified, but how do you unring a bell?

Around the circle, eyes darted right and left, Frances to Betty and back. Some stopped what they were doing; others hastened their task, as if ignoring the awkwardness would make it go away. Frances, who'd been rinsing a washcloth in her helmet, looked up. Her glasses were off; those around her were a blur. In a moment slowed by anticipation, all chatter stilled.

"Well," Frances finally said, considering Belanger's French name, "my people call it a *French* bath." There was a split second of uncertainty; then Frances burst out laughing with an exuberance not many had seen in her. The rest of the circle quickly joined in the raucous relief, none more enthusiastically than Betty.

Jews in the army during World War II sometimes found themselves targets of anti-Semitism; a small number of GIs thought Hitler was right to want to rid the world of them. Behind Frances's back, one captain in the Forty-fifth called her "The Kike." Once, Shoham lunged at an enlisted man who, with a certain snideness, had brought up Joseph's Jewishness, though another officer quickly broke up the would-be fight. But what

little friction flared in the Forty-fifth was usually between officers, notably nurses, and enlisted men whom those officers per-
ceived to be goldbricking.

Generally, Frances and the Jewish doctors experienced little prejudice. After all, it's hard to hate people who spend seven
days a week trying to save soldiers' lives.

By now, more than three weeks of daily twelve-hour shifts in
France had left a thick fuzz in the nurses' heads. Assembly-line
surgeries, lack of sleep, and moving every few days were beginning to take their toll. One night, Dottie woke up, shaking and
unable to sleep. Monty, a tent mate, turned on a flashlight.
Dottie was so stressed she'd broken out in hives. "I don't want to
face all this again," she told Monty, shaking her head back and
forth. "I don't want to get up."

Monty empathized. She couldn't forget one soldier whose
pain the doctors simply could not diagnose and who had died
amid the frustration. Still, she returned each day to the med
tents. So did Dottie and Frances and the rest. Nurses in the
Forty-fifth worked and slept themselves into an almost-mindless
rhythm. But they carried on.

As the day's heat intensified, Frances threw on her
fatigues—"Orglandes," that's where they were—and headed for
Shoham's mess tent to grab some chow before reporting to the
shock ward.

"Morning, Lieutenant," said Shoham, spooning a glop of
powdered eggs onto a tin plate for Frances.

"Happy Fourth of July, Joseph," she said.

Shoham smiled and shook his head. Of course, Frances, in
the midst of war, would be the one person to remember
Independence Day. She was apparently born patriotic, he figured.

In a corner of the mess area, two of Frances's tent mates, Elizabeth Powers and Christine Cox, argued about some trivial turf issue involving their respective space in the tent. Each nurse's "land claim" was an eight-foot-by-eight-foot swath and border wars were inevitable. As Shoham watched, Frances gently tried to broker a peace treaty but the bone-tired nurses weren't interested. Finally, Frances had had it.

"If you can't say anything nice," she said, "then don't say anything at all."

At times, nerves as taut as tent lines, nurses lashed out at one another, then made up in a moment, barely leaving a surface wound. "Like in all families," wrote Frances in a letter, arguments broke out. "But these were quickly forgotten." War, ultimately, did more to bring people in the Forty-fifth together than to tear them apart.

In fact, despite such occasional friction, despite the twelve-hour shifts and the lack of privacy and the pain of watching young men die and the setting up and taking down of camps . . . despite the taste bud–killing K-rations and the squatting on four-holers and the occasional pain-in-the-butt enlisted men, Frances, in a strange way, found an inexplicable peace in this life. Eerily, it echoed a poem she had written back in her prenursing years while she was struggling to find a place to belong.

> Gypsy how I envy you,
> Your open homes and skies of blue,
> Woman is as strong as man,
> And all belong to one big clan.
> Where you wish you pitch your tent,
> Forever forward you are bent,
> Hearts and hopes go with your men,
> You say one is as strong as ten!

With the stars and moon for light,
You dance your way into the night.

SOLDIERS FROM "Das Reich," the division that had massacred the people of Oradour-sur-Glane on the same afternoon the Forty-fifth Field Hospital had come ashore, reached the Normandy front in a somewhat piecemeal fashion. The first units arrived by mid-June, others not until early July. Six German soldiers from Das Reich deserted as soon as they arrived. On June 29, Adolf Diekmann, the commander who had ordered the massacre, was just north of Noyers, about twenty-five miles from the Forty-fifth's Second Platoon, when an Allied aerial attack erupted. He left the shelter of his dugout without a helmet and was killed by shrapnel that pierced his head from an exploding bomb. Other German soldiers who'd helped snuff an entire village on June 10, 1944, were already dead, too. But those still left alive were busy killing and wounding American soldiers, some of whom would wind up on stretchers at the Forty-fifth Field Hospital.

IN A CONVOY of trucks, jeeps, ambulances, and a 750-gallon water tanker, the Second Platoon rolled down the narrow, shell-pocked roads. Across cobblestone bridges and through gutted villages, they approached the seventh setup spot since landing at Utah Beach: Le Ruisseau. The nurses sat sideways in the back of ambulances and trucks, their presence sometimes triggering hoots and hollers from German POWs behind wire enclosures. Eyes often closed, the nurses tried to make up for lost sleep but made little headway, given the tank-rutted roads. Plastic packets of plasma jiggled in side panels behind them.

It was July 8, 1944. On either side of the Second Platoon lay burned-out tanks, overturned half-tracks, and American jeeps still smoldering from well-placed 88s, shells that traveled so fast that the explosion came before a soldier could hear their ghostly cries. Miles ahead, tanks chewed through the rubble of a village, tired infantrymen at their flanks. Once-thriving stone villas had been beaten into bare-walled remnants that looked like the back of stage props.

Nerves always tightened when the Forty-fifth approached a new town. At times, the unit would be the first to arrive after soldiers had liberated a village. With crumbled buildings still in flames from recent battles, truck windows often had to be rolled up to guard against the heat. So far, the unit hadn't encountered a wounded German left behind by his comrades with enough ammo and vengeance to go down shooting. But the fear never went away. German sharpshooters sometimes crouched in the bell towers of churches, coached to be looking for officer insignia on helmets and collars; a captain or lieutenant in the crosshairs of a German sniper was like finding a four-point buck in the scope back home—a highly valued prize.

We're a medical unit, rationalized some in the Forty-fifth. Off-limits. To which a less Pollyannaish sort would suggest bullets didn't seem to have the ability to recognize Red Cross brassards on anyone's arm.

By now, most in the Second Platoon had grown accustomed to seeing the bodies: the charred remains of some German tanker sprawled halfway out the hatch of the turret or a couple of bloody GIs lying lifeless amid the rubble. After a while, the carnage became so much a part of the landscape—some of the dead literally *were*, their bodies having been ground into muddy roads by tanks—that it bothered people less than it had in the beginning. And that discrepancy became bothersome in itself. To stop caring was, in essence, to cast aside the reason they were here. But war had a habit of grinding down any sense of nobility a doctor or nurse might have brought ashore.

As the convoy snaked toward the next camp, villages blended together with the sameness of their names. Oftentimes, French citizens would cheer, sometimes even kiss the hands of their "liberators." "Jeep! Jeep!" they'd yell. Just as often, though, Frances and the Second Platoon saw hungry people, shoeless children, and blank faces. And, occasionally, defiant looks from Nazi sympathizers and families who'd lost loved ones in U.S. air raids.

After feeding a throng of starving civilians, Shoham tossed an apron into a trunk. "We feed so many French we might as well start calling them our fourth platoon," he said to nobody in particular. Not far away, Frances held the hands of two little French girls, trying her best to help them forget the world of adults, even with a simple game of hopscotch.

Shoham's mess crew always led the way so they could get hot water ready for the surgical tent—and hot coffee for doctors and nurses—at the new site. The goal was to have the hospital up and running within one hour of the unit's arrival, though it took most of a day to travel from one place and get set up in another. Such was the case when the Second began making camp in a field near Le Ruisseau late on this Saturday afternoon, deep in the middle of the Contentin Peninsula and twenty-five miles east of Utah Beach.

Shoham pulled out his notebook, which now read like this:

10 March 1944: Landed at Cardiff England
10 June: Landed Utah Beach
11 June: Moved to Fauville
11 June: Moved to Audoville la Hubert
15 June: Moved to Fauville
17 June: Moved to Beuzeville au Plain
3 July: Moved to Orglandes

He added "8 July: Moved to Le Ruisseau" to the list, slipped the notebook back into his pocket, then started thinking about fixing dinner. The enlisted men went to work pitching tents. Done with that, they dug foxholes, trenched around tents in case of rain, and scooped out the ever-necessary latrine pit.

"Mail call!" barked a bone-weary private.

A letter had come for Frances. At first, the name on the envelope, "Catherine Bowler," puzzled her, then she realized it was from the sister of her tent mate, Margaret. Odd. Frances, leaning against a trunk, opened it and began reading. *Oh no!* The mother of the two sisters had died. Would Frances, when the time was right, break the news to Margaret rather than having her read it in a letter?

Frances didn't want to do it, but then, she'd done lots of things in the last eleven months that she didn't want to do. And who would want to find out a loved one had died by reading the news in the coldness of a letter? Later that day, before their shifts began, Frances broke the news to Margaret that her mother had died. In their musty field hospital tent, Margaret buried her head in Frances's embrace, the pain of one mother's daughter eased by another.

The death from afar personalized what sometimes had become routine. The nurses looked around. If a mother could die in a place far from war, then what of daughters who were in the thick of it? In a swath of rural France, twilight descended on the Second Platoon. The only colors that contrasted the greens and browns of the fields were the bold red crosses atop a half-dozen tents and a 100-foot red cross pegged in the field. They were symbols of safety amid a world that, here and now, seemed to offer little.

ACROSS THE SECOND Platoon's tent village, some dog-tired souls never heard it coming. By now, their ears had gotten used to the nightly air battles, the sky flashing like late-summer lightning, the roar of bombs. But others realized this was different, a more ominous sound, as if a plane had strayed from the heat of battle and was heading their way.

Pvt. William King, a surgical technician from Ohio, popped his head out of a tent. It *was* a plane, tilting to its side, on fire and out of control. Like a fireball, it bored through the darkness directly toward the Second Platoon's camp.

"Ge' down!" yelled King, at nineteen the youngest member of the Forty-fifth.

Frances and her tent mates—Elizabeth, Christine, and Margaret—scurried out of their bedrolls in the darkness. Others awoke, nerves drawn taut, minds disoriented, trying to comprehend a noise out of nowhere.

"Comin' right for us!" King yelled. "Foxholes!"

Frances and her tent mates instinctively drew together in a mass huddle. There was nowhere to run, nowhere to hide. In the Normandy night, what was now a wayward bomb tilted on its side, then veered slightly away from the camp. It dipped, crashed in a field not more than a bazooka shot away, then burst into flames.

Later, some from the Second Platoon ventured out to see the smoldering wreckage: a German bomber most likely shot down by American antiaircraft fire. Its two-man crew was dead. A few enlisted men waited for the inch-thick lug nuts to cool, then spun them off with crescent wrenches and later filed them into rings. A poor substitute for beetles or finely made German dental instruments, figured Shoham, but when it came to war souvenirs, to each his own.

The Allied breakout from Normandy came in late July, six weeks after the Forty-fifth had come ashore. It was called "Operation Cobra." On the morning of July 25, nurses and doctors in the Second Platoon heard a collective buzz grow like legions of locusts. Soon, some 550 fighter-bombers, P-47s, appeared in the sky, each guided by radio messages from forward air controllers riding in tanks at the head of armored columns. Upon command, the planes fired rockets and machine guns, and dropped 500-pound bombs. That wave was followed by 800 B-17 bombers.

The world below shook as if struck by a never-ending earthquake. Gaping craters pocked the hilly landscape. Smoke mushroomed from dozens of fires. One German commander lost seventy percent of his troops—dead, wounded, or crazed in what would go down as one of the greatest air raids in history. America paid a terrible price for its success: 111 GIs had been killed and 490 wounded, the highest number of casualties suffered in any single friendly-fire incident in World War II. But the bombing tore open a hole in the German lines and proved to be the turning point of the Allied invasion.

By mid-August, the small remains of the German army in Normandy were locked in a narrow pocket around Falaise, a hundred miles west of Paris. Hitler forbade retreat, trying to save face by subjecting his soldiers to a slaughter that was one of the worst of the war. Despite his orders, some 100,000 Germans surrendered on the spot. Still, the "Falaise Gap" was fish-in-a-barrel warfare. The landscape was littered with so many dead Germans that the few American soldiers who hadn't thrown away their gas masks put them on to keep out the stench.

The days grew warm as summer deepened. Frances and the other nurses, in sweat-soaked fatigues, mopped the brows of doctors doing surgery. Soldiers baked beneath woolen blankets. From time to time, the nurses fanned their patients, or gave them comic books so they could do it themselves. Enlisted men got crankier than usual, the heat making latrine duty worse than ever, if that were possible.

One day, Dr. John Bonzer was checking on patients in post-op. From the nearby surgery ward, a program called "Home News from the USA" droned from Dr. Hirsh's radio in the surgery tent. "Never thought I'd long for Normandy rain," Bonzer said to Frances, who was also working post-op.

"Or me for Boston's cold," she said.

She leaned over a wounded soldier and started to make small talk, but the soldier wouldn't answer the most basic question she'd ask. He was conscious. He lay naked beneath a blanket, a bandage on his chest, fear in his eyes. He was young, not yet twenty, and hadn't been shaving for long. Frances turned to Bonzer, a puzzled look on her face.

"He's German," said Bonzer.

Frances momentarily froze. Nearby, Shoham watched. Bonzer's Jewish tent mate didn't like the way the Second Platoon catered to German prisoners. Many wounded German POWs were more than happy to be under far better care and feeding than they'd get in their own outfits—and safe from the risk of being killed. One German POW said when the Forty-fifth reached Germany, his mother would cook the Second Platoon the finest meal they'd ever had. But Shoham didn't warm to such proposals. He'd once seen a German POW try to rip the IV tube out of a wounded American soldier. The Geneva Convention be damned; these were Hitler's henchmen who had been murdering his Jewish relatives. They deserved no favors.

Most POWs were compliant. But, like the others, Frances had seen the Jerries in the Second Platoon's medical tents who spit on nurses and panicked when a medic joked that the blood the German soldier was receiving was "*Jude Blut*—ha, ha, ha." And she hadn't forgotten the stories from the ghetto of Lødz, like the one about how the Nazis had once commanded a group of Jewish girls to clean a latrine—with their blouses. When the job was finished, their overseer celebrated by wrapping the blouses around the girls' faces and laughing heartily.

Bonzer walked away, then subtly glanced back. Frances looked into the eyes of the young German soldier. She then knelt next to him, raised her arm toward him, and dabbed his forehead with a cool rag.

ON AUGUST 6, the Germans began the deportation of the remaining 50,000 Jewish inmates of the Lødz ghetto. They were the last substantial group of Jews left alive on Polish or German soil, and they were now being crammed into railroad cars, up to 5,000 a day. They had been kept alive in order to work in factories set up to support the German war machine. But the German war machine was crumbling, so it was time to kill them.

The last transport left Lødz on August 30, having by now taken 76,701 Jews to Auschwitz, south of Lødz, and thousands more to another extermination camp, Chelmno, east of the city. Among them were all of Frances Slanger's relatives except one, a cousin named Franje, who was in hiding. Lødz, the first ghetto to be sealed back in 1941, was now the last to be liquidated. Slowly, train after train steamed away with all the Jews except for a scattered few hundred who'd found hiding places.

Within a week, the empty Lødz ghetto was as quiet as death itself.

SINCE THE BREAKOUT, the pace across France had dramatically increased and the number of wounded dramatically *decreased.* American field hospitals, like the troops ahead of them, were suddenly like some fleet-footed halfback who'd been trapped at the line of scrimmage—Normandy—then broken into the open field beyond. The Second Platoon, after spending most of June and July within thirty miles of Utah Beach, had traveled some three hundred miles in the three weeks since leaving Le

Ruisseau. From time to time, it linked up with the Forty-fifth's First or Third platoons; mostly, it operated alone.

It was September 3. To the northeast, the liberation of Belgium had begun the previous day. The Second Platoon had just hunkered down near the village of Bethencourt, about one hundred miles northeast of Paris, not far from Belgium's southern border.

Like nearly every other place the Second had stayed since leaving Normandy, the shops and houses of the village wrapped around a Catholic church. The spire of the structure poked some hundred feet into the air, topped with the same chicken weather vane to be found at nearly every other French church. Below, in the church's high-ceilinged sanctuary, a nook had been set aside to honor soldiers from Bethencourt who had died in World War I. Etched in stone were the names of the men who'd been killed in what was supposed to be "the war to end all wars." Twenty-six years before, these same rolling French hills had been strewn with the bodies of the fathers and uncles of some of the American GIs now fighting.

Churches did something to those involved in war. They were sanctuaries amid the insanity, touchstones of goodness buried in the rubble, reminders of the way things had been. Though it wasn't easy finding God amid the horrors of war, the Second Platoon's doctors, nurses, and enlisted men gathered for religious services when their schedules allowed. Chaplain Orlow Rusher was often too busy conducting memorial services and tending to the wounded to lead services, but groups sometimes gathered on their own. On Friday nights, the Jewish members of the outfit gathered for Sabbath services, Schwartz presiding. In the Jewish faith, ten people were required for a *minyan*, or quorum, to pray as a community, though when the Second couldn't always fill that requirement, a few non-Jewish nurses happily filled in.

Such services tugged at Frances's emotions, not only the thought of what she believed to be a kind and loving God existing amid the ruins of war, but of home. Of her mother and father and sister and nephews, thoughts tinged with sadness and a certain guilt. A portion of her $165-a-month pay was automatically sent home. Still, when given the rare moment to put things in perspective, she found herself wondering if she had been wrong to leave in the first place.

If spiritual forays triggered soul-searching, so, too, did the sound of Tiny Schwartz playing "Sentimental Journey" on a trumpet. On one afternoon, Schwartz had an audience of two: Frances and a wirehaired terrier named Penny. The dog and the horn were new acquisitions, having been bought in Paris a week before when some from the Second Platoon had gotten day passes to join the revelry of liberation that began August 25.

In Paris, amid hugs, kisses, and unending offers of wine and champagne—*Les libérateurs!*—Shoham had mailed home his first box of beetles to Ethel in the Bronx. And a group from the Second Platoon had chipped in to buy the dog as the unit's mascot. They named her "Penny," short for penicillin, the new wonder drug that was helping to save soldiers who surely would have died had the invasion begun only a few years earlier.

The sound of Tiny's trumpet in a French pasture soothed the afternoon. Nurses hung their wash on tent lines. John Bonzer, head propped on a bunched-up blanket, stared at the sky. Only days before, he'd gotten word that his father, "Chesty" Bonzer, the mayor of Lidgerwood, North Dakota, had died back home. Bonzer never got to say good-bye. Nearby, Maj. Herman Lord, the nondescript doctor who headed up the outfit, found his thoughts back in Detroit with his wife, Wilma. Other surgery-sapped doctors snoozed in fields splashed with buttery sunshine. The medical tent had a light load, not much beyond an enlisted man who'd been fishing a stream with hand grenades

---

and blown off his hand. It wasn't a particularly ethical way of angling, exploding grenades to kill fish, but then, war had a tendency of blurring the edges of ethics.

In the enlisted-men's area, Pvt. William King took a deep drag on a Lucky Strike cigarette and tossed in a couple of matchsticks to ante up in a poker game. Vincente Rivas, a twenty-two-year-old private from Socorro, New Mexico, rattled off a few lines in Spanish just to keep the opposition off guard. Among enlisted men, Rivas was the Second Platoon's poker king; King already owed him more than $50. Rivas was Catholic and the son of migrant workers. In the throes of the Depression, he had quit school after eighth grade to follow his father in the fields, honing his poker skills from camp to camp. Years and thousands of miles later, those skills were paying off.

Frances wrote a "V-mail" letter to Joseph Yanoff, her old Oneida Street pal who also was in France, serving with the Ninth Air Force. Others caught up on the last few weeks' issues of *Stars and Stripes*. Tiny Schwartz began a rendition of "The White Cliffs of Dover," triggering in the minds of some the sweet words, "There'll be love and laughter and peace ever after,/Tomorrow, when the world is free. . . ."

"Roosevelt says we're going to retake the Philippines," said Shoham, joining Frances and Tiny, "and that MacArthur is going to be part of the operation."

"Told you," said Frances without missing a beat. "He said he'll return. He will."

Shoham's attention was distracted by a butterfly. He watched it flit this way and that, then he returned to the paper. "When will the Germans fold up?" asked a *Stars and Stripes* headline. It was an intriguing question but not nearly as intriguing, some nearby soldiers thought, as the sultry photo of singer Dinah Shore, who'd arrived in France to entertain troops. Besides its pinup-girl photos and its "Prettiest WAC in the

ETO" feature, each *Stars and Stripes* edition included a feature called "An Editorial," in which some editor gently reminded the boys to keep fighting hard, keep their lips sealed and, with the VD rate skyrocketing after the liberation of Paris, keep their condoms on for sex.

Romance—and its less-refined relative, lust—took root in whatever meager plot war afforded. For Army Air Force pilots, red-crossed tents became the international symbol for American women, whether or not the nurses were available. Planes dropped notes or flowers by parachute, the men aboard asking the nurses for dates. A neighboring unit would send a scout to inquire about a handful of their guys coming for a visit. Shoham became something of a go-between. He'd throw together some sandwiches and coffee and chaperone a mixer.

Even the higher-ups saw value in the nurses beyond their service to the wounded. Once, while traveling between camp-sites, a chaplain from Boston chastised Betty Belanger for not wearing a dress. "We *must* raise the morale of the men," he told her.

The army wasn't naive. Back in March, when the *Florence Nightingale* had delivered the Forty-fifth to Cardiff, Wales, the first thing enlisted men got after coming down the gangplank was condoms. Though venereal disease was a huge problem as the war in Europe deepened, no cases among the Forty-fifth were reported during monthly checks. (Nurses weren't tested.) But then, the unit's monthly reports didn't show everything. They didn't show, for example, that a pup-tent liaison between a First Platoon nurse and an enlisted man—officially, nurses were supposed to be off-limits to enlisted men, period—had left her pregnant, and that she was sent back to the States as soon as word reached her superior. It was army policy—not that the fathers of those babies would be similarly booted.

Whenever the First and Second Platoons bivouacked

together, John and Sallylou rekindled their romantic embers. And Ed Bowen and Monty were talking about getting married soon, if they could get a superior to grant the request.

While on night patrol back at Fort Rucker in Alabama, Frances had come across a sleeping bag outside a tent that appeared to be inhabited by more than one person. With her moralistic antennae suddenly on full alert to a broken regulation, she shone a flashlight on the bundle, only to find a soldier fast asleep, a dog snuggled close. She smiled and walked on.

Hers was a black-and-white view of the world, where right was right and wrong was wrong, all of it tinted with a bit of Jewish legalism and Rockwellian idealism. By now, Frances's friendship with Isadore Schwartz had grown deeper. Though some enlisted men wondered if the relationship hadn't gone further, those who knew the two well doubted it. Isadore was, after all, a married man and Frances a respecter of virtue, even if she might have considered the possibility. Still, for the nurse who listened to the boyfriend-back-home stories from other nurses with a certain wistfulness, there had long stirred in Frances deeper urges to find that "one special one."

As Schwartz's trumpet soothed the harsh edges of war, Frances leaned with him against a battered trunk. She surveyed the beauty of France in a region that hadn't been ruined by war. Fields of green. Church spires. Stone farmhouses that looked so strikingly different from the row houses of Roxbury. Frances looked west, toward home, that place where she had sat on the roof beneath a star-studded sky and dreamed her dreams, often with pen in hand.

SHE CALLED the piece "And So At Last." She had written it sometime shortly before enlisting in the army. And it conveyed romantic longings embodied in the fictional character "Diane Macy," a nurse whom Frances placed on a long-overdue cruise.

At last Diane Macy sank happily into a deck chair, too excited to relax. Three days ago she felt as though she were going to suffer a cerebral hemorrhage unless something exciting happened soon. And so at last she made a break for it and here she was, on her way to New York.

Seven years without a vacation was a long time. Three years of study. Three years of living in the nurses' home . . .

Frances dutifully pointed out that Diane loved "every moment" of being a nurse. Nevertheless,

. . . Everything was wrong. She didn't feel happy. She had built a wall of reserve around her which at first the other nurses tried to break through and then gave up in despair. She had made few friends in her profession and did not have time to make friends on the outside. . . .

She suddenly realized that she wanted to get away. Away from the hospital. Away from the white-uniformed nurses and doctors. Away from pain and suffering and disgruntled recuperating patients. Away from hospital odors. She wanted to be surrounded by soft music, she wanted to wear soft pretty things and, above all, she wanted to find love.

Diane tried to read, but was drawn to music from the ship's ballroom.

An uncontrollable feeling of sadness enveloped her like a shroud. . . . She gazed at the swaying couples a little enviously. They belonged to one another. Where did she fit in? The only place she belonged in was the hospital.

At this point in her short story, Frances wrote that as Diane

looked at the floor—"the tears were very close to the surface"—
she was suddenly approached by a handsome man named David
Judge, who had "deep, gray, smiling eyes." He asked her to
dance.

> She began to feel so alive, so happy, so free. At last,
> something was happening. Instinctively, she felt that this
> stranger was going to change her entire perspective on
> life. This was where she belonged. . . .

His lips moved against her ear. He told her she danced
beautifully. They smiled at each other over a Coca-Cola. They
strolled the deck.

> He kissed her gently, passionately. She found herself
> returning each kiss. Her head felt light. She could reach
> out and touch a star. This was real, she knew it and felt
> it in her heart. . . .

Writing, Frances had long realized, was the best way to
unlock whatever small dreams she had. The hard part was making them actually come true. In her innocence, she could imagine being all that she was not. At times, she sketched drawings of
women with high cheekbones and long eyelashes. But if the
ships of her imagination featured lovers strolling the decks, the
ships of her real life were packed with immigrants and soldiers—
and, in time to come, coffins.

AFTER FIVE DAYS of doing relatively little, the Second Platoon
got orders to move out Friday, September 8, to a village called
Charleville. It would be the unit's last stop in France before
entering Belgium. The Germans had fled back to their country's

border some 120 miles to the east and were preparing one final defense of their homeland. After caravanning about seventy miles southeast, the Second set up its eleventh camp since leaving Utah Beach.

The sun slipped behind the rolling hills to the west. The Jews and their *minyan* fill-ins gathered for a Sabbath service in a field near the officers' tents, a band of ragamuffins pausing to remember. On a towel spread over an empty trunk, two candles flickered lightly in the gathering dusk, flanked by a bottle of wine and Shoham's best rendition of *challah* loaves, baked the night before. Tiny Schwartz stood behind the trunk. Nine people, including Frances, spread half-circle around him.

"*Baruch atah Adonai, Eloheynu Melech ha-olam, asher kid'shanu b'mitzvotav v'tzivanu l'hadlik ner shel Shabbat,*" began Schwartz. ("Blessed are You, Eternal One our God, Ruling Presence of the Universe, Who makes us holy with *mitzvoth*, and gives us this *mitzvah* of kindling the Sabbath lights.")

As the service continued and the sky above France faded from blue to black, the candles shone in the darkness, casting soft light on the war-weary faces of those who had gathered. For a moment, war seemed far, far away. Soon would come Belgium, then Germany, and, finally, perhaps, home.

CHAPTER 10

No more the glowing flowers of Spring
Enrich the sweet romantic dell;
Yet, ah, the tints of Autumn bring
A fading charm, a soft farewell.

—ANONYMOUS,
FOUND IN FRANCES SLANGER'S CHAPBOOK

The lull of the past few weeks ended as if the reprieve had been nothing more than a false spring. Near the German border, war returned to the Forty-fifth Field Hospital in a torrent of casualties. Doctors knew the push across northern Europe was getting old when they started recognizing the incisions of soldiers they'd operated on back in Normandy. Twenty-year-old wounded soldiers started looking forty. Their eyes had seen too much. Their bodies had endured too much. Their minds had turned to mush.

In Bastogne, the unit's first stop in Belgium, the Forty-fifth's three platoons converged, but there was hardly time for celebration. They treated a unit-record 2,822 casualties in five days. The carnage was the result of the Battle of the Hürtgen Forest, a confrontation so bloody that American troops suffered literally one casualty for every yard gained. It became known as "the place of death."

Rosh Hashanah and Yom Kippur, like the birthdays of nurses and doctors, got lost in the never-ending line of wounded. Finally, after the bloody week in Bastogne, came relief. In early October, the Forty-fifth's convoy left Bastogne and headed north, winding slowly through the wooded plateau of the Ardennes toward their next stop: Elsenborn, Belgium. Village after village celebrated them as long-awaited heroes. Homemade American flags fronted houses and shops, alongside the black, gold, and red of Belgian flags. The Belgians tossed flowers to the Forty-fifth, giving them jam and wine and hugs.

With no wounded awaiting them at their next stop, the unit took time to revel in the honor. Despite the language barrier, Frances befriended a Belgian family and posed for a photograph with the family matriarch. The woman sat in a chair. Frances, wearing a military dress and coat that made her look oddly formal given the Forty-fifth's gritty existence thus far, sat on the arm of the chair. Her arm was draped around the woman's shoulders: *Protector and protected.* The look on Frances's face offered the slightest hint of pride, as if this were one of those moments that made it all worthwhile. "Here we work so hard to save one life," she had written in contrasting the death of the young mother in Boston to the deaths of women and children in Europe. "*There* they work so hard to end life. . . ." Now, it was as if she'd played some small part in returning the virtues of life and freedom to a place that had been robbed of both.

On October 7, the same day Frances and the Second Platoon arrived in Elsenborn, Crematoriums II, III, IV, and V at Auschwitz incinerated 663 bodies. In Auschwitz II, 1,229 women prisoners were put to death in the gas chambers.

At 1:25 P.M., a group of female Jewish prisoners being forced to remove the corpses from the gas chambers to the crematory attacked an approaching SS guard with hammers, axes, and stones. They set Crematorium IV on fire and threw several homemade grenades. Machine-gun fire quickly squelched the uprising. Survivors barricaded themselves in a barn and prepared to resist. The SS men set the barn on fire, burning 250 people to death. That night, another 200 who took part in the uprising were shot to death.

An SS officer announced that if there were other such incidents, all prisoners in the camp would be shot. The five women who spearheaded the uprising were tortured in an attempt to divulge their accomplices. One woman, Roza Robota, smuggled out a message to the others: "You have nothing to fear—I shall not talk." None did. All five were paraded in front of the entire camp. And hanged.

ELSENBORN WAS a Belgian village so close to the German border that with field glasses, American officers could see Hitler's vaunted "West Wall"—the Siegfried Line—about three miles away. The village perched on a withered-grass plateau about thirty miles southeast of Liège, clumps of infant firs scattered amid the sagging barbed-wire fences. Elsenborn featured a few dozen houses, some with thatched roofs; five pubs; two schools; one hotel, the Zum Truschbaum; a sprinkling of shops; and a stone Catholic church, St. Bartholomeus, whose spire jutted skyward just across the street from the hotel.

After the Germans had swept into town in May 1940, en route to occupying France, they had promptly named the major east-west highway through the village "Adolf Hitler Road." Camp Elsenborn was located on the road. It had been a training facility lined with rows and rows of barracks but now lay vacant, the Germans having retreated weeks before. The just-arrived Americans wanted nothing to do with it; the Germans were notorious for leaving booby traps. Beyond that, it was an inviting artillery target for Siegfried-Line Germans who knew its coordinates well. That was among the few advantages of having been chased from an occupied country: The deposed troops knew the lay of the land they'd left.

The First Platoon bivouacked in Elsenborn on October 6, 1944. Frances and the Second Platoon arrived a day later, its fourteenth stop since Utah Beach. The Third Platoon set up about a half mile away. On orders from Major Lord, the Second's enlisted men set up the camp in a field near where Elsenborn's main east-west route, Adolf Hitler Road, intersected with its main north-south route, N647. Soon, a semicircle tent village had been established.

Frances found it refreshing to arrive at a village that hadn't been bombed, mortared, mined, or machine-gunned into shambles. Except for the occasional moo of a Holstein, Elsenborn was oddly quiet. Most of the residents had been ordered to nearby Malmèdy by the American soldiers. The few farmers who refused to go plowed nutrient-starved fields, all fertilizer having been taken by the Germans to make ammunition. A hint of smoke hung above the Forty-fifth's camp, the result of potbellied stoves that warmed officers' tents now that nights were growing colder. The stench of cow dung was more pronounced than it had been in France. The difference was that Belgian cows were alive.

At night, John and Sallylou resumed their romance in the officers' tent, snuggling at movies shown twice a week or whenever Special Services could get the balky French projector to actually work. By now, word had spread that in nearby St. Vith, Bob Hope, Marlene Dietrich, and Bing Crosby were entertaining troops, Crosby singing the already sentimental war favorite, "White Christmas."

Beneath mashed-potato clouds, the Forty-fifth caught up on news from *Stars and Stripes*. Boston Red Sox player Bobby

Doerr had left for the army in August, but had still won the American League's slugging title. And American troops had entered their first German city, Aachen, about twenty miles north of Elsenborn, just across the border. But war didn't weigh heavily on the unit in Elsenborn. Nurses washed their hair and gave haircuts and back rubs to others. Penny chased a black-and-white cat that Tex had adopted following the temporary exiling of Elsenborn's citizenry. Nurses and doctors posed for pictures that could be printed fast, Shoham having access to chemicals used to develop X-rays. For one pose, Tiny Schwartz stood with his arm around Frances, a smile on his face, his hulking frame so tall next to hers that he could have eaten a bowl of soup off her head. Frances, her hair tied up on her head and arms crossed, exuded a rare look of contentment, almost as if she were Diane Macy on the deck of a cruise ship.

"ON YOUR FACE on the ground, soldier!"

The shrill voice startled Shoham. He'd been sitting on a trunk outside the mess tent, stoking the fire used to heat up dish-washing water. It was, he realized, a Boston voice, with a pitch that could mean only one person.

"Well, hello, Lieutenant Slanger," he said.

"How about that back rub I promised you?"

By now, Shoham's back was bothering him more than ever. How could he say no to one of Frances's soothing massages? He stretched out on the grass, making sure to avoid cow pies, and enjoyed the finest back rub of his life. After a short nap, he turned to thank her but she was gone. Shoham mentally shook his head. Vintage Slanger, he thought: swooping in, making someone feel better, then disappearing.

• • •

DAYS LATER, as a group of nurses laughed in the distance, Frances sat against a tree outside her tent. Carefully, as if the letter in her hand would break if she dropped it, she unsealed the flap. They were rare, these messages from home, and even if she dreaded Mama's chicken-scratch English, she savored the letters as she would a piece of chocolate.

Down the row of tents, where the First Platoon was camped, the giggling and laughter from the group of nurses grew louder. Gradually, with a kind of schoolgirl excitement that war rarely fostered, the nurses formed a human chute outside the entrance to one of the tents. One of them started a tongue-on-the-roof-of-the-mouth drum roll. Others joined in.

"And now, from beautiful Elsenborn, Belgium, in the heart of the ETO!" announced Dottie to the entire camp, "we bring you the latest in war fashion, brought to you by the Forty-fifth's favorite model, Salleeeeeeeeee-lou!"

From across the camp, the heads of officers and enlisted men popped up as if an air raid siren had gone off, just in time to see Sallylou Cummings burst from her tent wearing nothing but a Nazi flag that she had stitched into a two-piece bathing suit. The swastika was located neatly on her compact rump. Applause erupted, liberally peppered with catcalls and whistles. Standing outside the mess tent in his apron, Shoham smiled broadly. Sallylou did some hip-swiveling runway struts, fluffed the back of her hair, and ended her performance with a gracious bow to the whoop-and-holler crowd.

John Bonzer shook his head and smiled. His girl had most of the Forty-fifth, and most notably *him*, firmly in the palm of her hand. He loved how she was full of life, in a way he'd never been. But if the incident had breathed a little life into a unit that had spent nearly four months dealing with despair, the lightness of the moment was lost on Frances. She stared at the letter, oblivious to all around her.

It was from her mother. *You must come home,* it said. *Your father—he has not much time. Please. Come now, dear Frances.* The news slammed her like some gust out of nowhere. And not only the idea of losing her father, but the idea of losing herself. Her father, now sixty-three, had been slowly dying for years. Frances knew his time was coming. What also jolted her was the idea of leaving the Forty-fifth, the wounded, the *mission.*

Come home? Didn't Mama understand? Didn't she understand what it was to see the fear in a broken soldier's eyes when the morphine wore off and he woke up, wondering where he was? Didn't Mama understand the thrill of seeing the first smile of some dogface whom she'd helped nurture back to life? To leave now was to fail.

Her officers' handbook was clear about priorities: "The citizen who dons the uniform as he enters extended active service leaves his chosen life behind him until the day of victory. . . . Within this space of time the service of the Country has the first and final claim upon his talents, his time, and his interest."

Frances got up and headed for her tent, past Sallylou and her fashion-show entourage. For years, Frances had felt herself no more in control of her life than the soldiers floating in the swells off Normandy, pulled here and pushed there by the whims of the waves. This was different. She'd fought to get here. She'd refused to be the proverbial straw in the river, carried here and there by forces beyond herself. And now she was supposed to simply give it all up and come home? How could she? The day of victory was yet to come. And, besides, she already *was* home.

Later in the tent, Frances lay on her cot. Darkness descended. Even an ocean away, she was, it seemed, still the fruit peddler's daughter, the nonstop "go-between" running errands for her parents whenever they asked.

This was triage time. *A system of priorities designed to maximize the number of survivors.* A system that, Frances realized, said *stay.* This, after all, was where the need was greatest, where the numbers beckoned. Or so said her head. But what about her heart—what did it say? How could she ignore the wishes of the woman who held her tight when the German soldiers burst into the Baluty flat in Lødz, the woman into whose arms she ran after she'd been let out of the cage at Ellis Island, the woman she almost lost one night back in Boston. . . .

THE SABBATH candles glowed in the row house windows as twenty-seven-year-old Frances hurried from the streetcar to the apartment complex on Wardman Road. It was early on a Friday evening, March 14, 1941, and the shift from day to night was almost complete. Suddenly, Frances stopped: A few blocks away, flames licked the sky. It was the Slangers' apartment building, engulfed in fire. Frances began running toward the inferno. *Mama!*

In the darkness, firemen scurried from trucks to the apartment, dragging hoses left and right. Police kept onlookers back. Flames crackled. Windows shattered. Frances stopped near the crowd that had gathered in the darkness. Her eyes darted from one person to the next, looking for that one face.

Where was she? Where were Sally, James, and the boys? And where were the other families in the unit—the Lemacks, the Mishkans, the Kengigsbergs? Frances shoved her way through the crowd, asking neighbors if they'd seen her family. They shook their heads sideways.

Mama!

She started for the burning complex. A Boston Rescue 2 firefighter grabbed her and held her back. Frances pulled against the firefighter's grip. She could save them. She knew she could. As a nurse, this was the lifeblood of her existence—to comfort the afflicted. To protect. To rescue. As a daughter, this was even a deeper duty: to save the woman who had saved her.

Mama, where are you?

At last, she saw a group of people emerging with a firefighter. It was her mother, wailing in her thick accent, and her sister and nephews. Sobbing. Coughing. But alive.

IN ELSENBORN, barely had the gravy cooled on Shoham's breakfast biscuits the next morning when word spread from one end of the mess tent to the next: Frances Slanger was asking for a ticket home. She had talked her way into coming overseas; now, she considered talking her way home. But this was different. Part of the reason Frances had convinced the brass to waive her Stateside restriction was because the U.S. Army Nurse Corps had awakened to the reality that it was woefully short on nurses, and Allied forces were about to invade France. In granting her request, the military wasn't being altruistic. It was being simply practical. Supply and demand. They needed her.

Request approved.

With Frances's request to return home, however, the brass saw no such outcome. Soldiers tired of digging biffy pits might be betting twenty francs that they'd be home by Christmas. And word had it that soldiers' winter wear was staying in England because the powers that be figured the war would be over before the cold and snow set in. But as Frances explained to Capt. William Poe about her mother's letter—probably with far less gusto than she'd used in arguing for overseas duty—the commanding officer knew German troops only a few miles away were digging in for a final defense of the Fatherland. And would do so with every ounce of resolve the Führer demanded. This war wasn't over yet—for the Allies or for Frances Slanger.

Request denied.

• • •

CONGRESSWOMAN Edith Nourse Rogers of Massachusetts took a most unusual trip for a politician in the fall of 1944, particularly for one who had once attended Madame Julien's finishing school in France: She flew to Europe, slogged through foot-deep mud, knelt by the side of wounded soldiers, and talked to GIs, doctors, and nurses. Rogers, sixty-three, had a keen interest in getting this war over fast. She was one of the few members of Congress to speak out against Hitler's treatment of the Jews. She had an intense interest in military issues in general, helping craft what would later become the widely hailed GI Bill of Rights. And she was an ardent supporter of women in the military; in 1941, she introduced the bill to create the Women's Army Auxiliary Corps.

Rogers had gone from being a "congressman's wife" to being far more in the last two decades. She had developed an interest in military nursing in 1917 when she accompanied her husband, John Jacob Rogers, of Massachusetts's Fifth Congressional District, to France and Britain during World War I. She had joined the Red Cross and worked at Walter Reed Army Medical Center in Washington. When her husband died in March 1925, she had yielded to pressure from Republicans and the American Legion to run for his seat and to continue supporting veterans. Saying that "the office seeks the woman," Rogers, then forty-four, won the special election, defeating a former governor with 72 percent of the vote, the first of eighteen lopsided electoral triumphs.

Now, Rogers was again pushing the boundaries, not just for women, but for politicians in general. "I wanted to give the mothers and fathers of my district and my state a firsthand account of how their sons are getting on and how their sons are being treated by the army and navy," she said.

On a trip that included fronts in Italy and Belgium, Congresswoman Rogers said she visited the Forty-fifth Field

Hospital. She may well have chosen the Forty-fifth because nearly half the eighteen nurses, and a number of the doctors and other officers, were from her home state of Massachusetts. She said she met a Lt. Frances Y. Slanger, whom she said was representative of the "heroic" nurses who "pooh-pooh the idea that they are heroic."

"I visited the tented hospital myself and found that the nearer they were to the front, the happier the nurses were in their service. They felt they were more needed and more valuable to the wounded there."

Later, in a speech to constituents back home in Lowell, Massachusetts, Rogers said:

> The wounded men receive wonderful care from the nurses. Due to a shortage of nurses in most of the hospitals, they are overworked. But they do not complain. Where there is work to be done they pitch in and and do it.
>
> Doctors and nurses are on the job twelve and fourteen hours a day, seven days a week. I met one high-ranking officer who was extremely bitter because one wounded soldier lay where he fell for six hours. That burst of righteous anger, I think, is one of itself significant of the excellent job our people are doing.
>
> Sometimes it is beyond my comprehension how the present number of nurses are able to accomplish so much. They deserve much praise, for they are performing miracles. . . .

AT THIS POINT, the Forty-fifth was supporting the First Army's V Corps, whose October 1944 reports said the Elsenborn sector was a "quiet sector." The bulk of the German forces in the area were defending the country's first city to be attacked, Aachen, to the northeast. In the First Army's daily intelligence reports, the V Corps entry elicited a monotonous litany of "nothing to note" references for the first weeks of the month. Forty-fifth Headquarter's Morning Reports noted day after day of "no change." The Forty-fifth's enlisted men, their hands chafed and calloused, didn't even bother digging foxholes; officers either didn't notice, or if they did, didn't question the departure from protocol. If anyplace in this war was safe, they figured, it was this.

Only one German Army infantry division, the Eighty-ninth, was operating opposite the village. It had suffered heavy casualties in action along the Siegfried Line in September. The division was stretched thin and wasn't carrying out offensive operations in the area. As a result, there were no American combat units operating between the Second Platoon's area and the German front line, just cavalry scouts on patrol to ensure that the Germans had not crossed into American lines.

In essence, the Forty-fifth was hunkered down in a waiting game: waiting for supplies from England, particularly fuel, to catch up with V Corps troops. Joined by American forces advancing from southern France, V Corps helped form one broad, 150-mile line mainly along the German border. Already, those in the Forty-fifth had begun getting paid in German marks. It was no secret what lay ahead.

The Siegfried Line that needed to be thwarted was a system of strong points that fortified Germany's western border more than two miles deep in places. Other than a last-gasp counteroffensive, the fortification was Hitler's last best hope to stop the Allied advance. The Third Reich had given up France, Belgium, and Luxembourg. It would not, the Führer vowed, give up its Fatherland, too.

The snaking Line consisted of an intricate series of defensive positions marked by pillboxes, bunkers, and trenches.

"Dragon's teeth," antitank barriers consisting of pyramidal concrete blocks with flat tops, awaited their armored prey. And thousands of S-mines, or "Bouncing Betties," fronted the line's western edge, in Belgium. When triggered, such mines popped about a yard in the air, then exploded. The force shot some 360 balls or small pieces of scrap steel sideways, the mine having a lethal range of twenty-two yards but able to wound a person up to 110 yards away. The object was to injure, not kill, because the Germans knew two or more men were required to carry a wounded soldier off the battlefield, which could quickly thin an enemy unit. Bonzer and the other doctors hated Bouncing Betties with a passion.

On October 10, four months to the day since the Forty-fifth had come ashore at Normandy, a U.S. reconnaissance platoon only a few miles south of Elsenborn was making its way east to the Siegfried Line. *Boom!* Amid a geyser of dirt, a severed leg and a plume of blood, a soldier screamed. The lieutenant leading the way had triggered a Betty. Four soldiers came to help. *Boom! Boom!* They, too, triggered mines. All lost legs. Such was the weapon feared more than any other. Mines, unlike firearms, were indiscriminate killers and knew nothing of the Geneva Convention that protected medics, doctors, nurses, and chaplains.

As the days in Elsenborn passed, Tiny Schwartz filled the quietness with Glenn Miller songs on his trumpet. Frances spent her time with him or by herself. Even at thirty-one—she'd had a birthday August 13 back in La Juillière, France—she was, in some ways, still the little girl in Boston looking for a rooftop where she could write. And so it was that in Elsenborn, where the mooing of cows and the rustling of wind in the fir trees could almost make a soldier believe the war was over, she would occasionally slip away to the edge of the camp to think and write and unleash her latent "gypsy" spirit. She knew of the restriction to stay in the immediate area, but "immediate area," she rational-ized, was a relative term. Finding a sanctuary in an infant fir grove next door wasn't like hitching a ride to Liège on a half-track.

As Sallylou cut John's hair outside his tent, they noticed Frances. Always lost in thought, she seemed to be, her head somewhere else. The days passed. The waiting game continued. Frances went to the woods to write and think. A week after arriv-ing, Sallylou and the First Platoon were ordered north to Heppenbach, Germany, to replace the Forty-second Field Hospital, the same unit they'd supported that first night in Normandy. The Second Platoon was now alone in Elsenborn, the Third Platoon dug in about a half-mile north, leaving behind an eerie quiet. From time to time, an American heavy artillery battalion that had established itself just west of the Second Platoon's camp shelled German positions to the east, over the field hospital's tents. But for the most part Elsenborn lay still.

Then one night it happened: An eighteen-man German scout team slithered past the light American patrols between the Siegfried Line and Elsenborn. This was the Germans' old neigh-borhood. It was dark, and American commanders thought it highly unlikely the Germans would send a patrol, especially such a large one, into an area of such military insignificance. A couple of jeep drivers learned otherwise. Their bodies were found in the morning, their jeeps missing.

"Those fire-eaters who accuse field hospitals of 'rear eche-lon' should have been there," an army reporter wrote in the 134th Medical Group's newspaper, about the Forty-fifth Field Hospital. "They'd have had some of the fire chilled out of their blood."

What the scout team was doing in Elsenborn, stealing jeeps, nobody knew. In fact, doctors and nurses of the Forty-fifth were never told that the enemy had been on their front steps, and left a calling card in blood. No need to create unnecessary fear.

AUTUMN CREPT southward across Belgium and from highland to lowland. Temperatures dipped. Nurses began putting IV bottles around potbellied stoves to warm up the blood for the few patients they had left. By mid-October, torrential rains began. Winterlike winds howled, particularly at night. Thunder occasionally rumbled in the distance, bolts of lightning searing the darkness. Pathways between tents turned to muddy bogs.

It was a Thursday, October 19, 1944. Twenty miles north, the First Army had broken through the Siegfried Line and was locked in a bloody battle to take Aachen, a city of 166,000 people. Fighting had gone on for weeks, much of it door-to-door, and Hitler had commanded his forces to defend the city at all costs. Casualties for both sides reached into the thousands—closer field hospitals than the Forty-fifth were doing the patching—and the city had been all but leveled.

In Elsenborn during a brief break in the weather, Major Lord tried to raise rain-dampened spirits by walking around with Penny in his arms. Vincente Rivas continued winning at poker. As rain pattered on the tents, the doctors, nurses, and enlisted men of the Second Platoon huddled inside, talking quietly. Frances and her tent mates took turns stoking the stove with damp fir twigs. Their fatigues and hair were permeated with smoke by now, the perfume of nurses who'd almost forgotten what Tabu or Intoxication even smelled like.

They skimmed through the latest stack of *Stars and Stripes*, now that they finally had time. In the October 9 issue, for the first time ever, the newspaper had handed over its daily editorial space to someone besides its own writers—Gen. Dwight Eisenhower, who wrote an open letter to German citizens outlining the ground rules now that Allied troops had entered their country. "We come as conquerors," he wrote, "but not as oppressors."

From the time *Stars and Stripes* began printing in France, July 4, it had made virtually no mention of nurses. Meanwhile, when a new boatload of WACs hit Normandy, the newcomers not only made headlines, but were listed by name. Once, a WAC wrote to the paper's "B—Bag, Blow It Out" column, complaining about having to wear leggings and not being able to buy perfume. A nurse responded, calling the WAC's complaints "childish . . . rest assured we spend our time in a much better way . . . taking care of our sick and wounded soldiers. . . ."

Though *Stars and Stripes* and the biweekly *Yank* magazine largely ignored nurses, Frances and her tent mates had read a number of letters—apparently in magazines or newspapers sent from home—in which GIs lauded nurses with gusto. But on this raw, rainy night, as she and her tent mates readied themselves for bed, Frances wondered aloud if such praise was valid. Wasn't such honor owed to the men in the foxholes, not the nurses in the tents? To the guys putting their lives on the line every day? To the wounded men who would more readily help the banged-up guy in the next cot than bellyache about their own plight? The four talked about the articles for a while, then the conversation veered elsewhere. But the letters had stirred something in Frances. Something deep.

That night, she and her tent mates crawled into their bedrolls amid a storm and distant gunfire, neither of which showed signs of slackening. Water dripped from the tent roof and simmered on the wood stove. Frances managed a few fitful hours of sleep, but awoke at 1 A.M. The sideways storm buffeted the tent as if it were a rock-anchored sack in a wind tunnel. Her tent mates slept on. Inside the stove, a damp piece of wood sizzled. Frances stared up at the darkness, her mind bouncing from this to that. But for some reason, it kept coming back to the GIs praising the army nurses.

As the storm raged outside, Frances slipped out of her bedroll. She turned on a flashlight, and began writing:

> It is 0200 and I have been lying awake for one hour, listening to the steady, even breathing of the other three nurses in the tent. Thinking about some of the things we had discussed during the day. The rain is beating down on the tent with a torrential force. The wind is on a mad rampage and its main objective seems to be to lift the tent off its poles and fling it about our heads.
>
> The fire is burning low and just a few live coals are on the bottom. With the slow feeding of wood, and finally coal, a roaring fire is started. I couldn't help thinking how similar to a human being a fire is; if it is allowed to run down too low and if there is a spark of life left in it, it can be nursed back. . . . So can a human being. It is slow, it is gradual, it is done all the time in these Field Hospitals and other hospitals in the ETO.

She paused, thinking of the earlier conversation with her tent mates. But the cold was distracting. She slipped back into her bedroll. Margaret woke up, then nodded off. It wasn't the first time she'd been awakened by Frances's nocturnal scribblings, which now continued.

> We had read several articles in different magazines and papers sent in by grateful GIs, praising the work of the nurses around the combat areas. Praising us—for what? I climbed back into my cot. Lt. Bowler was the only one I had awakened. I whispered to her. Lt. Cox and Lt. Powers slept on. Fine nurses and great girls to live

with . . . of course, like in all families, an occasional quarrel, but these were quickly forgotten.

I'm writing this by flashlight. In this light it looks something like a "dive." In the center of the tent are two poles, one part chimney, the other a plain tent pole. Kindling wood lies in disorderly confusion on the ground. We don't have a tarp on the ground. A French wine pitcher, filled with water, stands by. The GIs say we rough it. We in our little tent can't see it. True, we are set up in tents, sleep on cots and are subject to the temperament of the weather.

We wade ankle deep in mud. You have to lie in it. We are restricted to our immediate area, a cow pasture or hay field, but then, who is not restricted? We have a stove and coal. We even have a laundry line in the tent. Our GI drawers are at this moment doing the dance of the pants, what with the wind howling, the tent waving precariously, the rain beating down, the guns firing, and me with a flashlight, writing. It all adds up to a feeling of unrealness.

Sure, we rough it, but in comparison to the way you men are taking it, we can't complain, nor do we feel that bouquets are due us. But you, the men behind the guns, the men driving our tanks, flying our planes, sailing our ships, building bridges and to the men who pave the way and to the men who are left behind—it is to you we doff our helmets. To every GI wearing the American uniform, for you we have the greatest admiration and respect.

Yes, this time we are handing out the bouquets . . . but after taking care of some of your buddies; seeing them when they are brought in bloody, dirty, with the earth, mud and grime, and most of them so tired. Somebody's brothers, somebody's fathers and somebody's sons. Seeing them gradually brought back to life, to consciousness and to see their lips separate into a grin when they first welcome you. Usually they kid, hurt as they are. It doesn't amaze us to hear one of them say, "How'ya, babe," or "Holy Mackerel, an American woman!" or most indiscreetly, "How about a kiss?"

Frances thought of the hundreds of men she'd seen lying on cots from Normandy to Elsenborn, men she'd never seen before and would never see again. The flashlight was growing dim, the batteries nearly dead. Time, she realized, to finish.

These soldiers stay with us but a short time, from 10 days to possibly two weeks. We have learned a great deal about our American soldier, and the stuff he is made of. The wounded do not cry. Their buddies come first. The patience and determination they show, the courage and fortitude they have is sometimes awesome to behold. It is we who are proud to be here. Rough it? No. It is a privilege to be able to receive you, and a great distinction to see you open your eyes and with that swell American grin, say, "Hi-ya babe!"

She signed the letter, clicked off the flashlight, and fell asleep, her words, like everything else on this stormy night, lost in the darkness.

As FRANCES SLANGER slept, a landing craft thousands of miles and nine time zones to the east ground to a halt about 100 feet from the shore of a Philippine island, Leyte. A U.S. general wearing a starched khaki uniform, hat, sunglasses, and a determined look on his face splashed into knee-deep surf and strode purposefully toward the beach, along with an entourage of soldiers—and, of course, a photographer out front to capture the moment. Nearly three years after making his promise, Gen. Douglas MacArthur had returned.

CHAPTER 11

There are echoes of song that are sung no more, tender words spoken by lips that are dust, blessings from hearts that are still. . . .

—ROBERT L. TAYLOR,
FOUND IN FRANCES SLANGER'S CHAPBOOK

Well, what did he think? Sitting on a trunk in the mess tent, Capt. Joseph Shoham held up a "hang-on-a-sec" hand to Frances Slanger and continued reading the letter, trying his best to ignore his minions, the Rebels, who were arguing about dishwashing duties from breakfast. The smell of biscuits and gravy lingered with the outside smell of fresh cow manure, by now some soldiers unsure which was worse.

Shoham was wearing a well-smudged undershirt and unbuttoned field jacket. In one jacket pocket he had a things-to-do list, which included getting a few more bottles of whiskey for the enlisted men (he could manage that) and talking to Lt. Elizabeth Powers about her concern that patients weren't getting their food fast enough (she could blow it out her ear—until she got her orders in sooner). In another pocket he had a cupped napkin, a temporary container for a ground beetle he'd found outside the mess tent that morning and that was destined for his permanent collection back in the States.

"Well, should I?" asked Frances, eyes wide with hope. "Should I send it to *Stars and Stripes*?"

Shoham was lost in the words.

"*Well?*"

Shoham sniffed ever so slightly.

"Are you crying?" Frances asked.

On a landscape littered with the pitiful waste of war, Frances's words had touched something deep within Shoham, something he'd nearly forgotten he still had.

"Is it—?"

"Send it," he said.

"But what if they don't think it's good enou—"

"Send it, Frances," said Shoham. "Send it today."

Frances smiled as if this were such a rare moment that she didn't want to leave it. She pecked Shoham on the cheek and was off. Her tent mates—Christine, Margaret, and Elizabeth—heartily approved, adding their signatures to the letter.

Now, the day after finishing the piece, Frances wrote a cover letter for it. "We hope you will be able to find room for the enclosed article," she told the *Stars and Stripes* editors. "You see, we had many of these men as patients and that is the way we feel about it and them. For a change we want them to know how much we think of them."

The *Stars and Stripes* newspaper, since September 5, had operated out of the *New York Herald Tribune*'s office in Paris, where presses printed roughly 150,000 copies per week. In the "B—Bag, Blow It Out" column, a letters-to-the-editor forum, GIs had a chance to vent about this and that: *Why can't we get more cigarettes? Why no stories on our unit, which has done far more than those powder puffs you wrote about last week? When the hell are we goin' home?* And from WACs: *Why do some women get to take off their leggings and wear skirts? And why didn't we get credit for being the first WACS in Paris?*

Frances's letter was intended for this forum. She got the paper's address from her latest edition of *Stars and Stripes*, wrote it on an envelope, and gave the letter to a mail clerk. It was October 21, a Saturday, not that days of the week meant anything to anybody anymore. It was just another day of war—or at least began as such.

At Auschwitz, October 21, 1944, was a fairly typical day, too. The SS camp doctor conducted a "selection" in Transit Camp B-IIc. He sent 513 female Jews to the gas chambers.

In Elsenborn, rain fell hard. Finger-thick rivulets snaked their way through tents, the outside trenches having long since overflowed. Clouds shrouded the rural fields, muting greens, browns, and grays into a dark, dingy mass.

At 6 P.M., the Second Platoon gathered for dinner. What little light there was had already started to fade, the giant red crosses on the roofs of the surgical tents and in the nearby field soon lost in the night. Wind whipped tent flaps with increased vigor. Artillery fire sounded in the distance—by now so common that, like the whir of the generator, nobody much noticed.

After dinner, most headed for their tents, which fanned out in a semicircular arc, rounded at the top. Looking north, the mess tent was on the upper right, the officers' tent on the lower right, and the nurses' tent near the lower left. A few kerosene lamps dusted the interior of tents with light. Shoham stayed in the mess tent to prepare some French-fried potatoes that he planned to serve as a poker-game snack.

It was times like this, when he was alone and had time to think, when the war hit home deepest for him. And when the past returned so vividly. He and Ethel were coming up on their five-year anniversary. It had been nearly five years since they had up and eloped. They hadn't seen each other in almost eight months. He missed taking nature trips to Elmsford to collect frogs and turtles, studying the stars through a telescope in Van Cortlandt Park, and following the monarch butterflies as they fluttered across Staten Island every year. But more than all that, he missed his wife.

He'd met her at a nature camp in upstate New York, where he'd been a counselor. Now, as the rain pounded on the mess tent like pellets, he remembered how, a few weeks after that meeting, the apartment superintendent in the Bronx had knocked on the pipes to signal that Shoham had a phone call. It was his aunt in Mount Ivy, beckoning him to come visit. And when he did, there she had been—the fifteen-year-old girl he'd met at camp, Ethel, sitting on a bench, hugging her knees. Right then, he knew—just *knew* at age seventeen—that she was the one. Now, he thought of her back in their second-story apartment in Yonkers.

Suddenly, he heard something behind him in the tent. He turned. There was Penny, the wirehaired terrier, padding across the mud-grass floor. She stopped in front of Shoham and wagged her tail.

"Scared me, girl," he said, scratching her ears. "Good girl, Penny, atta girl."

In the arc of tents beyond, a poker game was being organized by the doctors, the ante pile heaped with French francs and German marks. Above the patter of rain and the diesel-fed generator rose the sound of a jeep, its tires splashing puddles and spraying mud. Two American soldiers in dripping raincoats arrived with the daily "poop sheet," a mimeographed update on troop movements in the area and on predicted casualties for the day to come. V Corps, which the Forty-fifth was supporting, reported "very little enemy 'arty' or mortar fire and very few enemy patrols." Virtually no casualties were expected the next day.

"We got Aachen," said one of the soldiers. "Finally."

Aachen, the first captured German city, would prove to be a turning point in the war. For the first time in five years, the people of Germany were lining Europe's roads as refugees. No longer was it the Poles or the Belgians or the French who were left homeless by war, but the people of the country that had foisted war on the world. Still, the victory triggered only a smattering of halfhearted clapping in the officers' tent. It was hard to celebrate the winning of a battle when you had so little perspective on what it all meant. To soldiers, a captured city meant time to move on and capture another city. The sense of winning such battles as a means to some glorious end had long since faded as the journey toward Berlin dragged on. And such victories were even less meaningful for doctors and nurses who were integral to the team but never actually "in the game."

The two soldiers left. Major Lord, as always, shredded the poop sheet lest it become an advantage to the enemy should the Germans somehow get hold of it. Lord poured himself a cup of joe and sidled up to a blanket-covered trunk on which the nightly poker game was about to start. John Bonzer tamped a fresh wad of Wilkie tobacco into his pipe, pulled the pipe lighter from his pocket, and puffed three times.

"Everybody in tonight?" he asked.

Bonzer was a quiet, serious man but poker, like Sallylou Cummings, made him feel young and careless. Besides, nothing like a game of five-card stud to take your mind off four months of sucking chest wounds. Hirsh joined the table, making it a foursome. Shoham would likely join later, they figured, after making the snack. He was always a welcome addition, not only because of his Bronx-based sense of humor but his ability to score whiskey in this area because he knew a little French and German.

"Five-card stud," said Bonzer and began shuffling the cards.

In a couple of pup tents joined together in the enlisted men's enclave, another poker game came to life beneath a lantern. The constant back-and-forth banter was distinguished by the occasional Spanish spoken by Pvt. Vincente Rivas. By now, Pvt. William King alone was into Rivas for $58. Back in Normandy, Rivas had shared one of the most horrific moments in King's war experience: One evening at dusk, the two had been thrown into temporary graves duty after they'd stumbled across the wreckage of an American plane. King was still having nightmares about that one, but in an odd way it had melded the two men together.

In the nurses' area, the scent of popcorn brought an instant back-home smell to a camp that otherwise reeked of wet canvas, cows, and mud. Gladys Davis Snyder, a dental officer from Frackville, Pennsylvania, and part of the Third Auxiliary surgical team supporting the Forty-fifth, began popping popcorn on a potbellied stove.

It was a little before 9 P.M. Down from Snyder's tent, Frances and her three tent mates settled in for yet another rainy night. The next day would at least offer something slightly different: fittings for new uniforms. Flashlight on, Margaret wrote home. Christine read by the light of a lantern. Elizabeth put the finishing touches on the wrappings of a few Christmas presents she had picked up en route from Bastogne, in a village named Malmédy, just southwest of Elsenborn; the gifts had to be mailed soon to have any hope of getting home by Christmas.

Frances sat on her cot next to Elizabeth, as usual, lost in thought. Of exactly what, her tent mates could only surmise, though by now they knew her well enough to surmise with considerable accuracy. Her mother's well-being? Her father's health? Her sister and her nephews? Probably. Or perhaps what had happened to all the nurses and guys she'd met back in Stateside training camps. Or the thought of autumn in Boston, how the speckled alder and Norway maples would now be bursting forth in one colorful last hurrah to herald the changing of the seasons.

And what of her own seasons? Thirty-one. Unmarried. Sitting in a tent in some cow pasture in Belgium, enduring weather only Noah could love. So much for those Diane Macy dreams of being the sweetheart of the cruise-ship ball, or, given the GI context, the sweetheart of even some ragtag *platoon*. Sallylou and John had each other. Monty and Ed were soon to be married. Isadore Schwartz had a wife back home and Margaret had taken a shine to a soldier she'd taken care of. But what about her? Who did she have? *What* did she have?

At work in a hospital tent, Frances could be as attuned to the moment as a concert pianist in mid-performance. But on nights like this, with no wounded soldiers to inspire her and no adrenaline to push her, she could easily be carried off in torrents of regret—the idea that, deep down, she was always the "also-pictured" person in the photograph. The never-quite-good-enough person, the guilt having grown thicker after she wasn't able to return home as her mother had requested.

But then, just as her inner struggles drove her deeper into this quicksand of remorse, the quiet thoughts would ease her out: The inspiration that she'd so carefully clipped and placed not only into some five-and-dime chapbook, but into her very soul. (Epictetus: "If you wish for anything which belongs to another"—even if that "anything" were the desire to be back in a general hospital where the nurses wore starched white dresses and drank nickel Cokes on their breaks—"you lose that which is your own."); the reminder, despite mud and blood and K-ration-triggered diarrhea, that life had something inherently good about it, as gloriously simple as a farm-fresh egg; and, above all, the plight of others instead of self. You could, she reasoned, lament having to "wade ankle deep in mud" or you could honor those who "have to lie in it."

Somewhere in the 200 miles between Elsenborn and Paris, in the back of an army mail truck, her letter with those words was en route to *Stars and Stripes* on this rainy October night. Bundled amid thousands of other pieces of mail, it was the handwritten fulfillment of all Frances Slanger hoped to be: Writer. Nurse. And above all, one who made a difference.

THE ARTILLERY SHELL screeched toward earth with the sound of a skidding freight train: thirty-two pounds of metal and high explosives designed to detonate with such force its concussion alone could kill. It hit near the edge of the Forty-fifth's camp like a burst of lightning and exploded in a hail of mud and shrapnel—jagged pieces of hot metal, some as small as fingernails, others as thick as a soldier's fist. A flash momentarily lit up the night.

Oddly, a quick outburst of nervous laughter burst from the tent where Rivas and others were playing poker, as if they thought this were no more than someone on uniform-burning duty having again forgotten to check for pocket ammo.

"Sounded like a shell," said Pvt. Larry Beaulieu.

"You must be hearing things," said King.

A second shell thundered down. Shrapnel blew sideways like a hurricane, ripping into tents, trees, and bodies. The laughing stopped.

"God, I'm hit!" yelled a man. "I'm hit!"

People fumbled to undo tent flaps, scrambled out of bedrolls, and staggered outside in foggy—and, in some cases, bloody—blurs of panic. Rivas tore out of the tent, sputtering something in Spanish, his cards still in hand. For the first time in the move across Europe, no foxholes had been dug because Elsenborn had been considered so safe.

"Where the hell should we go?" cried someone. "Where do we go?"

King, the nineteen-year-old kid from Ohio, sprinted into the pasture and down a gully. Suddenly, pain ripped across his thighs and he flipped forward; he'd run into a barbed-wire fence. Headed another direction, Rivas scrambled for cover in a garbage pit that had been dug. Amid the clamor, one thing was clear, even if the enemy's motives were not: The Forty-fifth Field Hospital was under attack. After months of treating the victims of war, the Forty-fifth was suddenly a victim itself. It was 9:20 P.M.

"G'down!" screamed Major Lord. "And cut the generators!"

Somehow, in the midst of the attack, Lord had the presence of mind to consider that the generators may have put a bull's-eye on the camp from an enemy position far closer than he'd thought. Someone flipped the Off switch, though the camp was still reeling in pandemonium—people yelling, rain pounding, and, every few seconds, another shell exploding. The sodden earth diffused some of the energy of the blasts—muddy soil beats dry soil in an artillery barrage—but in these frantic few minutes nobody was counting any blessings.

Adrenaline pumped. Smoke and rain and staccato words swirled amid the chaos. Frances and her tent mates donned their helmets and huddled together, arms around each other. Schwartz headed for the area where he'd heard the man's scream. Bonzer, who'd left his helmet in his tent, ran from headquarters to get it. Shoham, facedown in a swath of mud, suddenly remembered the pot of oil in the mess tent; one spark on that, he thought, and the whole place would be ablaze. He popped on his helmet, grabbed his flashlight, and began to run.

A thundering noise exploded and a geyser of debris shot into the air. Shoham was blown on his back. Nearby, shrapnel caught Schwartz in the hand and Pvt. Edward Knipstein on the bridge of the nose. Another scream pierced the night, this time a woman's.

Shoham lay in the field like a stunned bird that had flown into a plate-glass window. His eardrums pounded. Unsteady, he sat up and saw a light in the distance, but it was light with no context. Where was he? A penetrating heat bore into his right arm and, slowly, the fuzzy picture focused: the light was his flashlight some twenty feet away. This was war. He'd been hit. And he'd never felt more afraid in his life. He wanted to look at his arm but couldn't bring himself to do so. He wasn't sure it was still attached.

The world has no need for a one-armed dentist. In all the helter-skelter commotion, that's what Shoham thought in this moment. That, and if he were to survive, the only thing that would matter would be the love of his family and friends. He suddenly ached to be home. Ached for Ethel. He reached over and felt to see if he still had a right arm. He did. Soaked in blood, hot and seemingly growing more lifeless by the minute, but *there*.

Keeping his head low, he crawled through the mud to get his flashlight, stood up, and swept the beam across the field, looking for others who might be down. He saw Fred Michalove, who was searching for victims. He saw a huge figure, bent over in the darkness on hands and knees. It was Isadore Schwartz.

"Tiny, you OK?" asked Shoham above the roar of noise.

Schwartz didn't reply.

"Tiny, you all right?" Shoham screamed.

Schwartz stood up, holding his hand, his face grimacing. "Yeah," he said. "Just a thumb. Look for others."

Shoham scanned the field with the flashlight. Nothing.

Then, just as he was going to turn and head for the surgical tent, the light illuminated a brownish-red bundle in the distance, beyond the barbed-wire fence, near the garbage pit. Shoham stepped closer. Someone who'd been hit was lying facedown in the field, the rain and mud melding them as if one with the earth. Another someone—Michalove, it turned out—was kneeling over the body. The man down, Shoham realized, was Rivas, blood oozing from his mouth. A huge piece of shrapnel had torn through his chest, taking his heart and lungs with it. He was dead, his fingers still clutching a chilling reminder of how quickly life can turn to death: a pair of jacks.

Relentlessly, the shells continued pounding. An acrid haze hung over the camp. "Over here!" someone yelled. "It's Lord!" The major was lying beside a tent splintered with shrapnel. Shoham responded. He ran his flashlight beam from the major's head on down, then wished he hadn't. Lord's fractured left leg was bent back at a crazy angle. His right was worse. It had almost been torn off, raw flesh squeezing out in red and white bulges, blood burbling from fissures. He was breathing hard, his eyes glazed.

"Get 'em to surgery fast," said Shoham to a couple of privates who'd joined the search for the wounded, knowing the leg would have to go. Nearby, a nurse who'd tried to make a run from her tent was down. Bonzer ran to her side, joined by Schwartz, who was still trying to stop the bleeding of his thumb by wrapping it in his field jacket.

"Who is it, *Hunzeczech?*" yelled Shoham above the din of rain and commotion.

The nurse's face was splattered with mud. "Bowler, I think," said Bonzer, wiping away the mud on her face. In the darkness and rain, it was hard to tell who anybody was. He clicked on the metal pipe lighter he was never without. "No, wait—"

Another shell burst nearby. Bonzer and Schwartz shielded

the woman with their bodies. Mud splattered down. Bonzer took another look at the wounded nurse.

"Snyder!" he yelled. She was alive, but her thigh had been shredded by shrapnel.

"Need help over here!" yelled Bonzer. "I got this, Tiny. Go for others."

Fires crackled here and there. Now, from behind the camp, to the east, came flashes of light, explosions of guns, the whistle of shells passing far overhead. The American artillery battery, emplaced behind the Forty-fifth to the west, was returning fire to the east. That, mixed with the driving rain and waving beams of flashlights, only added to the ghostly sense of the surreal.

Amid the madness, Schwartz heard a faint cry from a female voice laced with panic. "Over here!" it came. "Over here!" He swept the beam of his flashlight back and forth. Veering toward the voice, he came upon a tangled mess of canvas, cots, tent poles, and laundry. Smoke poured from a wood stove that had tipped on its side. Schwartz's flashlight shone on a shattered French wine pitcher, what looked to be some sort of police badge, and a Star of David emblem.

Two nurses, Elizabeth Powers and Margaret Bowler, were sitting in the debris, vacant stares on their faces as coldly fixed as window frost. They appeared to have minor wounds. A third nurse, Christine Cox, was weeping.

"Over here," she called out between sobs. "Over here." Using a towel, she was trying to stop the bleeding of another nurse's stomach. It was Frances.

Schwartz bent over his friend in near disbelief. Shrapnel had slashed her stomach. She was hemorrhaging badly, the towel no less soaked than if it had been dropped in the Bay of the Seine. Rain spattered Frances's face and beaded on the dog tag that lay exposed on her field jacket. Her eyes, barely open, were hardly visible amid splotches of mud and a too-large helmet that, as always, was tipped cockeyed across her forehead. Nearby, her glasses lay in a puddle, the lenses shattered.

Shoham arrived, as did Frances's tent mates. Frances looked as if she were trying to speak, stopped, then reached deep within for the words she needed. Finally, with great strain, she opened her mouth.

"I . . . am . . . dying," she said.

Another shell landed nearby and lit up the sky. Schwartz looked around at the mass confusion, trying to will himself to act. He hesitated just a moment, reality now returning. He looked at Shoham's bloody arm.

"Get Bowler and Powers and yourself to the med tent," he said to Shoham, then turned back to Frances. The medical handbook be damned, he figured. If he moved her, yes, he might aggravate her injuries. But don't move her and they'd both be likely splattered by the next shell.

He leaned over Frances, dug his hands into the mud beneath her and winced when his torn thumb bent back. Like a human forklift, he slowly raised her. He cradled her limp body tightly in his arms like a father taking his sleeping child upstairs to bed, then headed through the downpour to the surgical tent some fifty feet away. Another shell screamed toward earth. It tore a hole in the field to Schwartz's left, splattering him with a sheet of mud and small pieces of shrapnel. He lumbered on through the rain, driven more by will than strength. The whistle of yet another shell approached the camp, but landed far off in the field. Finally, Schwartz reached the tent, Frances in his arms.

After firing some twenty rounds in a twenty-minute barrage, the German artillery ceased. Wounded cows bellowed in the field beyond. And the rain splattered on the roofs of whatever tents were still standing.

• • •

FRANCES SLANGER never had a chance. Bonzer knew it. Shoham knew it. Everyone knew it. After treating thousands of wounds, after seeing who lived and who died, those in the Forty-fifth got to the point where they just *knew* at a glance. Her face was already tinged a sickly green. But Schwartz wouldn't let her go. He pulled on rubber surgical gloves, wincing when the rubber bent his injured thumb. In a medical tent splotched with mud and blood, dripping with water from shrapnel holes in the roof, he furiously poured sulfa on the wound, then gave her a shot of morphine for pain. She faded in and out of consciousness, then opened her eyes and looked around at the handful of comrades who had gathered above her.

"Hang on, Frances," Schwartz said. "Hang on."

The fragment had sliced deep into her abdomen and to her spine. She desperately needed blood. Schwartz tried unsuccessfully to get an IV going.

"We could try a cut-down," said Schwartz. "Go to the ankle and give her blood." Shoham raced back to his dental kit for novocaine to suppress the pain of the cut-down, but when he got back he realized it was too late. Frances's breathing was getting irregular.

"Sit me up, sit me up," she said, believing that might help. For the handful of those in the Second Platoon who had gathered, it was a glimmer of hope. Schwartz helped her lean forward, but pain creased her face. She shivered. Her skin was cold and clammy, the look of someone slipping into shock. Her eyes grew wide and empty.

Facing her, Schwartz let go of whatever medical instincts that had ruled his days since Normandy and simply held her in his arms. He rocked her ever so slightly, those around inching closer in a oneness of grief illuminated only by flashlight beams.

Frances swallowed hard as if wanting to speak. "Oh . . . my . . . poor . . . mother," she said softly.

She stared upward. And then she was gone.

The surgical tent grew quiet in a way it had never grown quiet before. In the past four months, those in the Second Platoon had seen death in every way imaginable. They'd heard the last words of dozens of soldiers. They'd just seen an enlisted man, Rivas, with his heart torn out and an officer, Lord, with a mangled leg that was being amputated in the next tent over. But nothing could have prepared the nurses and doctors for losing Frances Slanger.

"Shalom," whispered Schwartz. He eased her down. Christine, now more composed, helped him drape a blanket over her tent mate's body. Dr. Isadore Schwartz walked outside in the rain and dark, fell to his knees, and sobbed.

LATER THAT NIGHT, after what sounded like more counter-battery fire from the American artillery position emplaced to the west of the camp, the Second Platoon gathered for an impromptu service for Slanger, Rivas, and Lord, whose condition was critical. Schwartz presided but nobody felt much like talking, including him. Prayers were offered. Hugs exchanged. It was past midnight. The rain had stopped and a silence hovered as if the sky were holding its breath.

Bonzer blinked back tears. It didn't matter that he'd grown up in rural North Dakota and Frances Slanger in Łødz, Poland; that he was a doctor and she a nurse; that he was a Catholic man and she a Jewish woman. What mattered, he thought, was that they'd been soldiers together in war, fighting to save the wounded. And now she was dead. It was bad enough watching young men die whom you didn't know. It was worse, he now realized, losing people you'd worked beside while trying to save those young men. He watched as, one by one, those in the Second Platoon walked off to be by themselves. Rivas's poker pals went to his tent, packed up his gear, and divided up his cigarettes among themselves.

In the next few days, whenever Joseph Shoham thought about losing Frances Slanger, his wounded arm began throbbing. Some enlisted men, such as Sgt. Charles Willen, who'd thought Frances Slanger something of a spoilsport, found themselves humbled by her death. They wished they'd treated her better.

Two days after the attack, Lord died from his wounds. Snyder, the dental officer with the thigh wound, recovered. She was sent to an evac hospital and, eventually, home to America. Penny, the Second Platoon's mascot dog for the last two months, disappeared during the October 21 shelling. She was never seen again.

PLUM-COLORED CLOUDS spit flakes of snow to the ground that awaited the body of Frances Slanger. Three days after the attack, dressed in an olive-drab uniform and wrapped in an army blanket, her body was lowered into a grave at the U.S. Military Cemetery at Henri-Chapelle. The cemetery was about twenty miles northwest of Elsenborn, in Belgian countryside where farmers were fixing fences that had taken months to put up but had been snapped in seconds by rumbling tanks.

The cemetery had no grass. No marble. No gardens. It was simply a stark splotch of hillside dirt that had become mud with autumn giving way to winter. Six weeks before this cemetery hadn't existed. Now, more than 2,000 graves of American soldiers dotted the hillside. Rows and rows of white wooden crosses, along with a sprinkling of Star of David markers, stood in stark contrast to the brown soil now being dusted with snow.

Frances was buried in Grave 20, Row 1, Plot T. Stenciled on the Star of David marker was her name and service number, in black:

FRANCES Y. SLANGER
N-752108

She had died at age thirty-one, the same age her mother had been when she had given birth to Frances in Łødz. Two American flags, each about a foot high and stuck in the ground on either side of the marker, hung in solemn stillness. All was quiet, save the sound of shovels slicing into almost-frozen dirt, the occasional whinny of a horse, and the sporadic thud of guns to the east, near the Siegfried Line.

Rabbi Sydney Lefkowitz, an army chaplain, said a few words to the handful of soldiers who'd gathered, none from the Forty-fifth, which was too far away to attend the service. He offered quiet Hebrew prayers, then looked to the sky. On this day, October 24, 1944, snow would blanket the western front for the first time since the Allied invasion of France.

A young black soldier stood near the grave, raised a bugle to his lips, and played taps. The mournful song once again reminded the farmers nearby that another soldier had fallen in the quest for freedom—Belgium's freedom and countries beyond. A few farmers stopped their work, doffed their hats, and stood facing the cemetery, darkened figures silhouetted against a landscape now draped with a whiteness that softened the jagged edges of war.

For weeks now, they had heard the sound of the bugle again and again. It blew not just to honor a fallen soldier, but to honor somebody's son, somebody's husband, somebody's father, somebody's brother. And now, for the first time since the landings at Normandy, somebody's daughter.

CHAPTER 12

Drop a pebble in the water; just a splash and it is gone;
But there's a half-a-hundred ripples circling on and on,
Spreading, spreading, from the center, flowing on out to the sea
And there's no way of telling where the end is going to be . . .

—ANONYMOUS,
FOUND IN FRANCES SLANGER'S CHAPBOOK

It was twilight on a late-October afternoon, cold enough out-side so the hide-and-seek kids on Roxbury's Homestead Street could see their breath and pretend they were smoking cigarettes. Inside, eight-year-old Irwin Sidman was listening to *The Green Hornet* on the family's Philco radio. From the kitchen, the smell of pot roast infused the cramped second-floor flat.

Irwin's mother, Sally, was fixing dinner, though in recent weeks she'd told Grandma Slanger she didn't know how much longer that would last because she was nauseated by even the sight of food. She was expecting her third baby. Grandma Slanger was asleep in a stuffed chair in the living room, Irwin's three-year-old brother, Jerry, still down for an afternoon nap.

A young man in a Western Union uniform came to the door. Was she Sally Sidman? With a sister somewhere in war-torn France, she didn't want to be. Not when being handed a telegram. But when the man left, she forced herself to open the message, which said:

MRS. SALLY SIDMAN
126 HOMESTEAD ST.
ROXBURY, MASSACHUSETTS
THE SECRETARY OF WAR ASKS THAT I ASSURE YOU OF HIS
DEEP SYMPATHY IN THE LOSS OF YOUR SISTER SECOND
LIEUTENANT FRANCES Y SLANGER REPORT RECEIVED
STATES SHE DIED TWENTY ONE OCTOBER IN BELGIUM AS
A RESULT OF WOUNDS RECEIVED IN ACTION.
                                    THE ADJUTANT GENERAL

Sally pursed her lips together, closed the door, and leaned back against it. She cupped a hand across her eyes, sliding it slowly down her face, unleashing tears. She looked at her mother, asleep in the chair, and wanted to leave her just as she was, at peace.

"Mama," she said softly, bending down beside her, then, when not waking her, louder: *"Mama."*

Eva Slanger awoke. She looked at her daughter's damp eyes, then at the telegram in her hand. Slowly she began shaking her head sideways.

"No . . . *no* . . . NO!"

Sally's subtle nod came with great reluctance. Eva's face contorted into twisted pain, tears welling. "Not Frances . . . Not my daughter . . . Not my baby Freidel!" Eva buried her face in her daughter's embrace, repeating Frances's Yiddish name over and over, just as she had when the doctors at Ellis Island had taken her away. Only this time her daughter wasn't coming back.

Irwin saw it all but didn't understand. All he knew was that something bad had happened. Aunt Frances was never coming home again.

• • •

Somewhere in Luxembourg, just south of Belgium, Pvt. First Class Millard Ireland leaned back in one of the thousands of foxholes that pocked the rolling hills. It was November 10, 1944. His M-1 Garand lay across his lap as he browsed the November 7 issue of *Stars and Stripes*. Sporadic gunfire boomed far to the east, near the German border. Ireland thumbed through the paper. Roosevelt was a solid bet to win an unprecedented fourth presidential term. On the Eastern Front, the Soviets—the other side of this Allied vise—had stormed the suburbs of Budapest. And, oddly, the usual staff-written editorial was missing. In its place, a headline piqued his interest: "A Nurse Writes the Editorial" it said.

Ireland began reading: "It is 0200 and I have been lying awake for one hour . . ."

The GI's casual interest deepened; he straightened the paper and read on. "With the slow feeding of wood, and finally coal, a roaring fire is started. I couldn't help thinking how similar to a human being a fire is . . ." By now Ireland was engrossed in the words of this army nurse, whoever she was. By the time he got to the end, his eyes were moist.

Frances Slanger's piece had not only been published in *Stars and Stripes*, but had been given top-of-the-page display— not as a letter to the editor but as a guest column on the editorial page. Since the newspaper had begun publishing in the ETO July 4, only one other person had been allowed the guest-editorial space: Gen. Dwight Eisenhower. Across northern Europe, on land and at sea, more than 100,000 issues with Frances's editorial had been delivered to soldiers, sailors, and airmen. But like the *Stars and Stripes* editors, none of the readers had heard what had happened to her after she'd mailed the letter.

Later, Ireland scrounged a pencil from his pocket. "To the nurse who wrote the editorial," he began. "The S&S editorial of November 7 was such as to bring a lump to a dog-face's throat. It is more than touching to be told you are made of good stuff by somebody who ought to know, with such obvious sincerity as that of 2/Lt Slanger." Continued Ireland:

> We men were not given the choice of working on the battlefield or the home front. We cannot take any personal credit for being here. We are here because we have to be. You are here merely because you felt you were needed. So, when an injured man opens his eyes to see one of you lovely, ministering Angels concerned for his welfare, he can't help but be overcome by the very thought that you are doing it because you want to.
>
> . . . You could be home, soaking yourselves in a bathtub every day, putting on clean clothes over a clean body and crawling between clean sheets at night, on a soft, springy mattress. Instead, you endure whatever hardships you must to be where you can do us the most good.
>
> I'd better stop now because I'm getting sentimental, but I want you to know your "editorial" did not change, but only confirmed, my deep respect for you modern Florence Nightingales. If the world had a few more people like you in it, there wouldn't be any wars.

In an old stone farmhouse not far away, Pvt. Lynwood R. Zebley and others in his unit huddled around a fire built to stave off the November chill, taking turns reading the nurse's piece. As it passed from man to man, the room grew quieter and quieter. Like Ireland, Zebley, too, wrote a letter. So did lots of other soldiers across northern Europe. Not a handful of them. Not dozens of them. *Hundreds* of them, tired soldiers who stopped in the middle of a war to say thanks to a woman who they didn't even know.

"I have finished reading the editorial for the third time," wrote Sgt. Paul Cooney of the 502nd Parachute Infantry of the 101st Airborne Division, somewhere in Holland. "It is by far the best editorial ever published in S&S. This is the general opinion of my whole platoon. . . ."

Not far away, in Holland, Pvt. J. A. Marfin read the article that had been recommended to him by a buddy. He'd never been so impressed with anything he'd read. Carefully, he tore it out and placed it in his field-jacket pocket, next to his heart.

The "Boys from the 1st Division" wrote: "She and the other members of her Corps are the living Angels of Mercy, having a life of Hell under fire and going through their daily tasks of relieving the pain of the wounded and sick. Never complaining of their own hurts and loneliness, but always ready and willing to listen and comfort the wounded on the lines. I would suggest that a citation be conferred on Nurse Slanger and each and every other nurse under fire from China to Germany."

On November 9, Orlow A. Rusher, the Forty-fifth's chaplain, wrote to Eva Slanger from Belgium. He knew what the GIs across northern Europe did not. While expressing his sorrow, he pointed out how highly regarded Frances had been, not only by her own platoon but by other units the Forty-fifth had encountered. "One unit," he wrote, "gave her a lovely write-up in their division paper. They acclaimed her as 'Honorary Division Sweetheart.' "

IN PARIS nearly a week later, *Boston Herald* reporter Catherine Coyne, a portable typewriter in one hand, stuffed a few francs into a cabdriver's hand and hurried into the headquarters for war correspondents, the Hôtel Scribe. Coyne—at thirty-seven, tall and slender with dark hair and blue eyes—had just learned the news: The nurse who'd written the editorial for *Stars and Stripes*, the nurse who everybody was talking about, was dead. And she was from Boston. Coyne would break the news to America.

On Thursday, November 16, 1944, a rainy day one week before Thanksgiving, Bostonians awoke to Coyne's front-page article. It was just below a story on Gen. Douglas MacArthur.

Roxbury Girl First U.S. Nurse To Die Under Nazi Fire in West
Lt. Frances Y. Slanger Paid Touching Tribute In Stars and Stripes to Courage of GI Joes

By Catherine Coyne
(Boston Herald-N.Y. Times Wireless)

Paris—Lt. Frances Y. Slanger, 126 Homestead Street, Roxbury, Boston City Hospital graduate with a First Army field hospital, was killed in action Oct. 21 by shell fire, I learned today. She was the first American nurse killed in action in this theater.

Seventeen days later, ignorant of her death, Stars and Stripes printed as an editorial a letter she wrote to the editor paying tribute to the wounded American soldier and assuring him nurses regarded it "a privilege to be able to receive you, and a great distinction to see you open your eyes and with that swell American grin, say, "Hi-ya babe."

Though primarily a tribute to the fighting man, there shone through the warmth, humor and sincerity of the letter-editorial a spirit of selfless service that motivated this American nurse's work at the German front [sic]. It was one of the most widely talked about editorials in the serviceman's paper. . . .

In a follow-up article to her initial report on Frances's death, Coyne wrote that the editorial "better describes the spirit of front line hospitals than articles by war correspondents."

In the days to come, Teletype machines in newsrooms from Boston to Los Angeles clacked with the Slanger story as wire services spread the news across the nation. Families heard it on living room radios, talked about it in nickel-a-cup coffee shops, and read it in their local newspapers. Once "the fruit peddler's daughter," Frances Slanger was now known as "the nurse who wrote the editorial."

"Wounded don't cry, nor does dying nurse" declared the headline in New Orleans's *Times-Picayune-States*. Some papers put Frances's story on the front page. Dozens of others chose to forgo their regular editorial column and let Frances's piece say it for them. "In the place of our leading editorial, we print below a poignant letter . . ." wrote the *Florence* (Alabama) *Herald*. "We wish this letter could be reprinted in every newspaper in the United States. We wish a copy of it could be handed to every civilian who hesitates when asked to buy a war bond or begins thinking up excuses why he can't buy more. . . ."

In Holland, Pvt. J. A. Marfin, the soldier who had carried the Slanger article in his pocket since the day he first read it, leaned against a stone wall in the late-November darkness, weary from another day at war. Soon, a fellow GI approached him. It was the same buddy who had pointed out the Slanger editorial to him a few weeks before. He was carrying another copy of *Stars and Stripes*, the just-out November 22, 1944, issue. He handed it to Marfin without a word, but with eyes that said he knew something he wished he didn't.

The headline jolted Marfin: "1st ETO Nurse Killed in Action." He looked below the mug shot of a woman: It said, simply: *Frances Slanger.* Marfin looked his buddy in the eye, then bowed his head in grief. How, he wondered could someone so good—so courageous—be dead?

The top-of-the-page headline capped a ten-inch story about her death. Since *Stars and Stripes* had begun publishing more than four months before, it was the first time the newspaper had run a picture of an American woman that wasn't a cheesecake shot or a "prettiest-WAC-in-the-ETO" shot. The photo was published not because of how the woman looked. It was published because of what she had done. And how she had died.

The story, whose author had interviewed members of the Second Platoon, included most of the details of the *Herald*'s story, but added more: "Her friends said that Frances Slanger knew she was dying, but uttered no word of complaint. Her chief concern was of the grief her death would bring to her family in Boston."

Milton Zola, Frances's childhood friend who had wound up with the 552nd Antiaircraft Automatic Weapons Battalion in Germany, broke down after reading the news. So did others. Marfin tucked the second article next to the first, in his pocket, then wrote a letter to *Stars and Stripes.* "We have all lost a real, true friend when we lost Lt. Frances Slanger," he wrote, "but she died as she had lived, a hero." Sgt. George W. Fritton, an air gunner with the Army Air Force's 647th Bomb Squad, 410 Bomb Group, wrote this letter from France, signed by eight other airmen:

Inspiration is difficult to discover. We discovered it. Amid the roar and thunder of war emerges at one time or another the genuine, worth-living-for thoughts of a human being. Only few people can put it on paper—but all of us have that singular, infinite thought deep in our minds and hearts. Frances Slanger put it on paper—so overwhelmingly beautiful yet so much from the heart. She captured the distinguishable characteristic of human love and understanding which has become so latent in our speedy world. She portrayed modesty in the nth degree—looking for no praise, but gathering the hearts of millions of GIs into her possession and then losing them. Losing them in this life to her memory, but retaining them in that unknown world to come.

Frances Slanger is a great woman. We say *is* because her memory in our minds will linger steadfastly long after the final gun is fired in this war. Why? Because Frances Slanger pointed out the only genuine rule for peace on earth: human love and understanding.

By the time the stream of responses had trickled dry, Frances's piece had triggered more letters from GIs than perhaps any single editorial ever printed in the *Stars and Stripes* during World War II. And the response symbolized a bittersweet truth about her: The woman who had never found that "one special one" had, in fact, found many. It was as if she'd come to the dance by herself and still managed to be chosen queen of the ball, or as Chaplain Rusher had pointed out: *Honorary Division Sweetheart.*

Many of the hundreds of men who lauded her in letters did more than express sorrow. They suggested, in some cases *demanded*, that something be done to honor her: Publish her letter and GI responses on every front page of every newspaper. Issue a citation for every ETO nurse in honor of Frances. Erect a memorial, but do *something*.

Some didn't wait around. The 117th Infantry Regiment of the 30th Infantry Division passed a hat and quickly had a "sizable collection" for a memorial. Second Lt. Aubrey J. Olham, who flew a P-38 Lightning in the ETO, got an artist pal to paint Frances's picture on the side of his plane. "In Memory of Lt. F. Slanger, U.S.A.N.C.," it read.

Lt. Eugene C. Bovee believed Frances deserved more. "It is my opinion that there would be no finer way to honor this courageous woman than to name after her the best and finest hospital ship yet to come off the production lines," he wrote. "I believe, too, that aboard that ship, in a position readily legible to all, should be a plaque bearing the words of the letter she wrote to the American wounded. No other epitaph could do her more honor than her own words."

IN ROXBURY, the last leaves of autumn skittered down Homestead Street as if warning of the approaching winter. The windows of apartments on the street were sprinkled with blue-star banners, meaning a soldier, sailor, or airman on active duty had family there. In a window of the Slanger/Sidman flat, the blue star had given way to gold, meaning the family had lost someone in the war. Eva Slanger found herself knotted in pride and grief.

One day, she received a letter from a woman named Louise Ostermann of Liège, Belgium, who wrote that she had been placed in charge of Frances Slanger's grave. To honor those who had liberated their land from the Germans, the Belgians had begun what they called the "Godfathership of the Graves of the Dead American Soldiers." Citizens adopted graves of the deceased, vowing to "visit the grave of your soldier regularly, to decorate it with flowers whenever possible and to give you news and a sort of faith echo across the seas concerning the last resting place of your son, brother, fiancé, husband or friend, Frances Y. Slanger."

It bothered Eva that the person keeping watch over her

daughter's grave—in Hebrew, a *shomer*, or guard—assumed Frances was a man. The army did the same thing at least three times. So did Massachusetts Governor Leverett Saltonstall, who, ironically, had just lost a son himself in the South Pacific. What bothered Eva more, however, was Frances's body being so far away. Her daughter's body was seven miles from the border of the same Germany whose soldiers were murdering her people, and had not been buried according to Jewish tradition.

Like many parents who lose children, Eva was grieved not only by the idea that she would never see her daughter again, but that her daughter might be forgotten. Months before, she had tried to get Frances to come home, but to no avail. Now that her worst fears had come true, she at least wanted Frances's body home, lest her daughter's memory blow away in the wind.

Meanwhile, the response continued. *The New York Times* published an editorial that lauded Frances and nurses like her. *Newsweek* wrote about her. In Washington, D.C., Congresswoman Edith Nourse Rogers honored Frances with words of praise before Congress. People across the country clipped the Slanger story from their hometown newspapers and sent it to Eva, a few addressed simply to "Mrs. Slanger, Boston, Mass."

"One day the name of 2d Lt. Frances Y. Slanger will be linked in the annals of the Army Nurse Corps with the same reverence universally accorded Florence Nightingale," wrote Kent Hunter of the *Boston Evening American*.

While Slanger's story spread far and wide, it dug particularly deep into the hearts of Boston's Jews. The Jewish War Veterans established the Frances Y. Slanger Post No. 313, the first such all-woman organization in the nation.

Hollywood gossip columnist Hedda Hopper substituted her usual entertainment theme with a letter sent from "Spec" McClure, a former colleague of hers who was now serving with the army in Belgium. He wrote about "a dead girl whom I never knew but whom I, doubtless, along with countless others, felt I knew." He described Frances as "a model of a selfless devotion, a humanity, and an integrity one thinks extinct."

> She wrote as a GI Jane to a GI Joe deeply involved in a bloody business called war, asking not for understanding, expecting no mercy, but giving to her limits in both.
>
> And we knew there wasn't a false word in the letter. . . . We knew it for our world, and we grinned in appreciation, knowing that we read the letter of a girl already dead, and her words fixed beyond alteration. They were sealed with her blood. . . .
>
> During this war, as both civilian and soldier, I've seen ideals trampled in the mud by those who most profess to uphold them. I have seen this too often to have much faith left. And I have seen, as all who make an honest effort must, a thousand forms of betrayal and stupidity. And in weariness I have told myself a thousand times nothing remained to believe in—that the ancient enemies of mankind, greed and ignorance, were too great for our mortal strength to conquer. But now I know that this is not altogether right.
>
> For somewhere in the sordid, selfish, shameful business that makes up most of our petty lives there is a nobility that will not perish. . . .

In Frances Slanger, McClure saw the manifestation of such nobility. What he saw, amid a war rooted in Hitler's greed, fear, and ignorance, was something that months of combat had doused but that Frances's words had rekindled: hope. For more than four months, Frances had given it to individual soldiers. Now, her letter had given it to them all.

Honor for Frances continued. On the day after Christmas, 1944, Frances's posthumous Purple Heart was presented to Eva. In January, a New York–based radio show, WABC's "We the People," presented a program on Frances, hosted by Hollywood actress Joan Fontaine. Frances's sister, Sally, was invited to take part.

"Tonight," said the announcer, "Joan Fontaine brings you one of the most moving stories to come out of the war—a story of an army nurse that surpassed anything Hollywood has ever dreamed of. . . ."

A Sgt. Sidney Leyman wrote to Eva from Belgium to say he'd visited Frances's grave at Henri-Chapelle and that it was in fine condition. "We treasure [Frances's] memory," he wrote, "because she did her work, regardless of race, color, or creed, and that's what we are fighting for."

With the letter to Frances's mother, Leyman included a photograph of a flower he'd left at the grave of Eva's daughter. It was a *myosotis*, more commonly known as the "forget-me-not."

As JANUARY 1945 deepened, Allied troops supported by the Forty-fifth and other field hospitals continued fighting the bloody Battle of the Bulge after a surprise German counteroffensive. The days had grown so cold that when the Second Platoon's doctors made an incision in a man's stomach, steam sometimes hissed out. Back at the cemetery at Henri-Chapelle, deepening snow crushed and buried the flower left by Sergeant Leyman. As Frances's buddies trudged farther from Belgium and deeper into Germany, the snow climbed higher and higher on the Star of David marker at the head of her grave. Soon, it threatened to obscure her stenciled name altogether.

• • •

On January 18, 1945, the last Jews still alive in Lødz, Poland—Frances's cousin Franje perhaps among them—were hiding in a cellar when they learned the Germans were looking for them. If found, the Jews would be ordered to dig nine large graves—each for a hundred people.

The next day, those in hiding heard boot steps outside. They'd been found, these last few Lødz Jews who thought they'd somehow escaped the Nazi wrath. The sound of boots grew louder, then stopped outside the cellar's entrance. Water dripped from the cellar walls. Slowly, the door handle turned. The door swung open. The Jews cowered in a corner. As they looked up, they saw, in the dim light, soldiers in uniforms they'd never seen. They were not German soldiers who'd come to kill them. They were Russian soldiers who'd come to liberate them.

"Today, at 11 A.M., the long-awaited moment arrived," Jacub Pozanski, one of the Jews, later wrote in his journal. "We are free!"

Germany's last-gasp counteroffensive in the west stunned and decimated a number of American divisions. But, ultimately, it failed. Soon thereafter, while by himself and without a weapon, Capt. Joseph Shoham stumbled across four unarmed Germans. The enemy soldiers looked at him. He looked at them. He'd never seen the enemy so close—and he was outnumbered. He felt the dry-mouth fear of Elsenborn. Suddenly, the Germans raised their arms in surrender.

"*Kamerad!*" they said. "*Kamerad!*" Imagine this, he thought as he nervously steered them back to camp: Joseph Shoham, a Jewish mess-hall boss, having Germans surrender to him!

Meanwhile, Monty Montague had been shipped home. Wearing paratrooper boots, she had married Ed Bowen at Thanksgiving in Bastogne and had gotten pregnant after a

Christmas Eve liaison with her new husband. Pregnant nurses weren't allowed to serve, thus the ticket to the States.

By spring, as Allied troops began pushing toward Berlin alongside thousands of German POWs walking beside the roads, the war was essentially over. But the horror wasn't. One day in April, Allied troops began inhaling a stench of death like no other they'd smelled: the Bergen-Belsen concentration camp, which had earlier been liberated by the British.

The Americans were stunned. They'd had no idea this had gone on. They had seen the anti-Jew sentiment, the *Die Juden sind unser Unglück* scrawlings ("The Jews Are Our Misfortune") on the stone walls of German towns. But until they saw the football-field-long stack of bodies, they'd had no idea.

The victims—most dead, some all *but* dead—were people from across Europe. Doctors. Students. People who'd had *lives*. Some 35,000 unburied bodies were strewn and stacked at Bergen-Belsen; 30,000 prisoners clung to life, most walking skeletons. American soldiers bent over and vomited. Wept. And looked to the heavens.

Atrocious as it was, Shoham realized, this is why the Americans had come. In a sense, their arrival was a case of "too little too late." But if it was true that President Roosevelt, who died only days before the grisly discovery, was too passive in rescuing the Jews, it's also true that the Allied liberators had ultimately come. And with their arrival, the mass murders stopped.

ON APRIL 28, the Forty-fifth was America's forward-most hospital unit when Russian and U.S. units linked for the first time, shaking hands, posing for pictures, and drinking champagne along Germany's Elbe River. "Today we have the most happy day in our lives," said a Russian major in broken English, a happiness, Sallylou Cummings later surmised, due partly to the hungry Russians helping themselves to the Forty-fifth's ample food supply.

Two days later, in his underground bunker in Berlin, Adolf Hitler stuck a pistol into his mouth and shot himself to death. His last will and testament placed "sole responsibility" for the millions who'd died in war, and in the death camps, on the Jews. His body was burned. No one offered a eulogy.

On May 7, Germany surrendered unconditionally to the Allies. After five years, eight months and six days of fighting, the war in Europe was over. What some remembered most vividly about Victory in Europe (V-E) Day were the lights. For the first time since the landing at Normandy, with the fear of air raids over, lights shone at night. And yet in the aftermath of war lay hundreds of shattered villages such as Oradour-sur-Glane, millions of soldiers' graves, millions of refugees with no homes to return to, six million dead Jewish people, and nearly that many other dead "nondesirables."

When the war ended, the Forty-fifth Field Hospital Unit was in Pilsen, Czechoslovakia, south of Poland. In 331 days, they had traveled 600 miles from Utah Beach. The unit that had begun with 226 people finished with 173. Though only three had died in combat—Slanger, Rivas, and Lord—the Forty-fifth had lost forty-nine people to wounds, illnesses, and pregnancy.

Since landing at Utah Beach, the Second Platoon had picked up and moved thirty times. The Forty-fifth's three units had treated 4,950 patients and performed a thousand major operations. The doctors and nurses had seen 223 people die while in their care. Tiny Schwartz left for Europe weighing 250 pounds; he now weighed 180.

At Passover, as Shoham walked along the streets of Pilsen carrying matzo under his arm, a man stopped him and asked him something in Yiddish. *"Entshuldikt, uber bist du a Yid?"* Yes, said Shoham, he was a Jew. The man smothered him with a hug. He and his wife, the man said, were the only remaining Jews left in

Pilsen. All the others had been taken to the camps. All the others were dead.

Flyers with General Eisenhower's written words of thanks were passed out to all: "That task which we set ourselves is finished. . . . No praise is too high for the manner in which you have surmounted every obstacle."

In the weeks to come, the Forty-fifth relaxed, swam, played tennis, played baseball, and partied. John, Sallylou, and others made plans to visit Paris and the French Riviera. Meanwhile, stars Jack Benny and Ingrid Bergman came to entertain the Forty-fifth because of a connection with one of the men in the outfit. Sallylou, not surprisingly, got her picture taken with Benny, his left arm draped around her as if they'd been dating for years. At one point, Benny said he'd play for the Forty-fifth if anyone could find him a violin; someone did and the master musician performed. Later, someone asked Tiny Schwartz to play his trumpet, but he declined. He hadn't played since Elsenborn.

The Forty-fifth split up. Its members went their separate ways, few to ever see one another again. Before climbing into a truck that would take him to Marseilles, France, where he'd sail for home, Shoham spotted something crawling on a cobblestone street. He bent over and coaxed it into his pillbox. It was a beetle he didn't have, something called a "tiger." A slight smile creased his face as he stuffed it into his pocket and continued on his journey home.

One for the road.

NEAR LIÈGE, BELGIUM, in fields beyond Henri-Chapelle Cemetery, apple blossoms opened their rosy fists after winter's siege. At the cemetery itself, an American flag fluttered at half-staff. It was May 30, 1945—Memorial Day, three weeks after V-E Day.

Victory's price stretched out on the gentle dirt slope:

17,500 white crosses and Stars of David representing American soldiers who'd given their lives in World War II, Frances Slanger among them. Charles Sawyer, the U.S. ambassador to Belgium, stepped to a makeshift podium and, through rimless glasses, looked out at an audience of mainly soldiers, not the least of whom was General Eisenhower.

"I speak to you today as an American," began Sawyer, fifty-eight and trim, his white hair flecked with gray. "I am talking to all of you—those who are here alive and who will return home, and to those thousands of Americans who are here in the sacred soil of Belgium and who never will go home."

Sawyer, a former World War I major from Ohio, lauded Belgium and England for their efforts in the war. He praised America despite its flaws. He affirmed democracy. He honored Winston Churchill. And in three sentences, he remembered the late President Roosevelt who, "exhausted from his great effort of leadership, missed by only a few weeks the magnificent spectacle of complete victory over the enemy."

Sawyer paused. "And now," he said, "I wish to pay tribute to a woman." He then proceeded to talk about 2d Lt. Frances Y. Slanger for the remainder of his speech; in fact, more than a third of his fifteen-minute talk was devoted strictly to her. Later, he would personally decorate her grave with a wreath. For now, he read a good portion of her letter. He explained how she had died on the rainy night of October 21, 1944. And he ended his speech with these words:

> Her friends said that she knew she was dying but uttered no word of complaint. She lies here in Henri-Chapelle with the rest of you who will not go home.
>
> The GIs to whom your letter was written cannot talk to you, Frances Slanger. They who could talk are not here; they are scattered all over the world—millions of

them—and so for them and for all Americans I say this to you in answer to your letter:

We thank you for the things you have said about the GIs; they are better said by you than by any other. If there is in heaven and in our hearts a special shrine for those who have given the most and the best, it is held sacred for the American nurse . . . her courage, her strength, her endurance, and her unfailing hope are the essence of the things which have given us this victory and which we believe will never die.

There was a momentary pause, then applause erupted, some from war-weathered soldiers whose eyes were now wet with tears. It was the first time anyone could remember hearing clapping at the cemetery at Henri-Chapelle, much less clapping that grew louder and stronger and wouldn't seem to end, the same kind of clapping that, three weeks later, rose from the Todd-Erie Basin Shipyard in Brooklyn, New York.

In a ceremony awash in red, white, and blue bunting, a 632-foot ship was being commissioned. It was a snow-white vessel emblazoned with four red crosses and a thick, green stripe at mid-hull. Stern first, it slid down the wooden way and splashed into the flood tide of Upper New York Bay. Cheers broke out. Workers tossed hard hats into the air. Flashbulbs popped.

Because of the desperate need for a ship like this, nearly four thousand men and women, the largest American contingent to ever work on such a project, had been called to transform it in six months' time. The vessel originally had been an elegant Italian cruise ship, named for the goddess *Saturnia*, and featured a Pompeiian swimming pool, a monumental staircase, and lavish marble. But it had now been refitted into a more utilitarian ship, whose purpose was far more important than the coddling of the rich. It was a hospital ship, bound for France, where it would bring America's wounded home from the war. It was the largest and fastest such ship yet to come off the production lines—the equivalent, in size, of three large hospitals.

It recently had been named by Gen. George C. Marshall, the U.S. Army Chief of Staff, in honor of a fruit peddler's daughter. The refurbished ship was called the *Frances Y. Slanger.*

FRANCES SLANGER'S life was forever marked by the comings and goings of ships at sea. And so it was that on July 1, 1945, a sunny and hot Sunday, the ship set sail for Cherbourg, France, not far from Utah Beach, where the Forty-fifth Field Hospital had once landed. Every doctor, nurse, and enlisted man who came aboard was given a handout with the story about the woman for whom the vessel was named—about the letter she'd written, the death she'd died, and the legacy she'd left.

With tugs at her side, the ship eased out of Brooklyn's Erie Basin, a blast from her foghorn announcing her presence. Then, slowly, the bow of the *Frances Y. Slanger* cut boldly through the blue chop toward The Narrows. She steamed south, away from Ellis Island and the echoes of a little girl crying in a cage. Away from the Statue of Liberty and its call to the huddled masses. Away from the land Frances Slanger had loved, cherished, and defended. Turning east after plying Lower New York Bay, the ship grew fainter and fainter as it headed into the open sea. And, finally, she disappeared, leaving behind a wake that spread toward distant shores.

Like ripples from a pebble dropped in the water.

EPILOGUE

JAPAN'S surrender on September 2, 1945, ended World War II. David Slanger, after spending nearly six and a half years in Jewish Memorial Hospital—and suffering from pneumonia, bronchitis, and emphysema—died on April 17, 1947, following a heart attack. He was sixty-five.

Five months later, Eva Slanger received a letter from the U.S. Army. Like other parents of those who'd died in the war, she had the option of having her loved one's body returned to America. She wanted that. So did sixty percent of those whose sons had been buried at Henri-Chapelle.

In early October 1947, in the Belgian port city of Antwerp, soldiers began loading 6,248 sealed, metal caskets aboard the *Joseph V. Connolly*, a U.S. Liberty ship similar to the one Frances and the Forty-fifth had sailed on from England to France. These were to be the first American war dead to come home.

One casket was chosen to remain in Antwerp's town square, surrounded by four guards, to honor all the soldiers whose bodies were being placed on board. The casket was Frances Slanger's.

All night long, before the ship was to depart, the four soldiers stood watch over Frances's coffin. The following morning, it was carried aboard the *Connolly*. Then, escorted by the U.S. destroyer *Vesole*, the ship headed west through the English Channel and home to America.

In New York, on October 26, an unseasonably warm day, America waited. It was a Sunday. Fifty empty railroad cars were lined up at the Brooklyn Army Base, ready to disperse the bodies, most to hometowns across America. In downtown New York, people started gathering by the harbor at daybreak. A crowd of hundreds became a crowd of thousands. People waited patiently for the ship's arrival. At 9 A.M., the *Connolly* broke through the haze outside The Narrows, a funeral wreath on her forepeak.

As the *Connolly* arrived in New York Harbor, scores of servicemen and dockworkers stood at attention, most wearing black mourning armbands on their left arms. A twenty-one-gun salute was fired from the First Army headquarters on Governors Island. By order of President Harry Truman, American flags flew at half-staff.

Pier 3, from which many of the dead had said their good-byes before leaving for Europe, was draped with all forty-eight state flags, each paired with an American flag. Before reaching that dock, though, the *Connolly* stopped at Pier 61, where a single casket—it wasn't revealed whose—was brought ashore and carried in solemn procession down the Fifth Avenue of Heroes.

Church bells tolled. Men doffed their hats and saluted. Those who lined the streets, some 40,000, watched in quiet reverence until a woman's edgy voice broke the silence. "Where's my boy?" she shouted. "Where's my boy?"

Ultimately, all 6,248 caskets were unloaded at Pier 3, where they would leave for their final destinations by rail. On November 14, Frances's body arrived at Boston's South Station. Eva was there, along with Sally and Sally's husband, James Sidman. Beyond the family, sixteen members of the Lt. Frances Y. Slanger Post No. 313, the first all-woman post in America, were also on hand.

Frances's body was taken to Stanetsky Funeral Chapel in Dorchester, where it lay in state that evening for three hours. Slowly, the line of people walked past: family friends, schoolmates from the High School of Practical Arts, nurses from Boston City Hospital, and veterans from both wars who paused to salute their comrade. A handful of people from the Forty-fifth paid their respects, only one doctor among them: Isadore Schwartz.

Elizabeth Powers, wounded in the same blast that had killed her tent mate, knelt at the casket. Her eyes were misty. "Hello, soldier," she whispered.

On November 21, a cold and overcast Sunday, a horse-drawn caisson—the same caisson that had carried President Franklin Roosevelt's body to its final resting place in Hyde Park, New York—carried Frances's flag-draped casket to the Crawford Street Synagogue in Roxbury. An honor guard from the Lt. Frances Y. Slanger Post walked alongside the casket, as did members of the Boston City Hospital Class of '37, wearing hospital whites, and a group of Gold Star mothers who'd lost children in the war. People in overcoats, hats, and gloves quietly watched the procession. Eva Slanger, standing near the synagogue, wept quietly.

More than 300 people crowded into the synagogue. Later, an estimated 1,500 people attended the committal service at Independent Pride of Boston, a Jewish cemetery in West Roxbury. Boston Mayor John B. Hynes attended the burial, as did Col. Florence A. Blanchfield, superintendent of the Army Nurse Corps in Washington, D.C., and other dignitaries.

Frances's grave was next to where her father's was and where her mother's would someday be. Soldiers removed the flag from the casket, folded it, and presented it to Eva. Then, one by one, as is Jewish custom, people stepped forward to place a small rock at the base of the headstone, a symbol of their being present at the grave.

The lower part of the gravestone read:

LT. FRANCES Y. SLANGER
BELOVED DAUGHTER AND SISTER
KILLED IN BELGIUM OCT. 21, 1944

Below, her name had been inscribed in Yiddish—*Freidel Yachet Slanger.* Only in death, it seems, was her full identity understood. For most, it was the first time they'd known what the "Y" had stood for in her name. "May her soul be bound in the bond of everlasting life," read the Hebrew inscription.

The headstone was etched in a pattern of flowers on both sides, framing the symbol of the Army Nurse Corps. The upper part of it included a line from Frances's letter to *Stars and Stripes:*

U.S. ARMY NURSE CORPS
"THE WOUNDED DO NOT CRY,
THEIR BUDDIES COME FIRST."

At last, the casket was lowered into the earth. A squad of riflemen fired a volley in her honor. Soldiers saluted. And finally, just as in the stark ceremony at Henri-Chapelle in Belgium, a lone soldier raised a trumpet and played taps.

Eva's daughter was finally home.

BOSTON'S SOUTH END, where Frances grew up, and Roxbury, where she lived before leaving for the Army Nurse Corps, now bear scant resemblance to the days when the Slangers lived there. The original apartment building Frances lived in was bulldozed to make room for a new office for the *Boston Herald* in 1957. The High School of Practical Arts for Girls, where Frances had graduated, closed in 1954 and Abraham Lincoln Intermediate School in 1976. The last graduating class of Boston City Hospital's School of Nursing was the Class of 1975.

In 1951, the corner of Angell Street and Blue Hill Avenue was named "Frances Slanger Square." Today, the corner is an iron-barred commercial strip. The sign has been gone for decades.

Though others in the Forty-fifth said Frances was "forever writing" in her five months in Europe, the last known piece of writing that's been found of hers—other than the letter to *Stars and Stripes*—was a farewell piece she wrote in January 1944 for the *Camp Gordon Cadence* in Georgia. It ended, "Thanks!—For a grand stay."

AFTER ITS LAUNCHING in June 1945, the *Frances Y. Slanger* hospital ship made five trips to Europe and back, bringing home the wounded from the war and, on at least one return trip, taking German POWs from America back to Europe. On its final voyage, it sailed from New York to Bermuda to assist another hospital ship that had run aground. With its hospital duties finished, the ship assumed its original name, *Saturnia*, and, in 1946, was released to its Italian owners. The ship was scrapped in La Spezia, Italy, in 1965.

IT WAS RARE for the Germans to fire on a medical facility on the Western Front during World War II, even accidentally. The shell that killed Frances Slanger was most likely fired by a 105mm gun belonging to the 189th Artillery Regiment of the German Army's Eighty-ninth Infantry Division. But the shell was almost certainly not intended for the Forty-fifth Field Hospital. The unit had been in reserve at Elsenborn for more than two weeks without incident, and the German formation had been opposite the entire time.

The Forty-fifth only became a target when an American heavy-artillery battalion moved in after the medical unit had already set up its camp. From time to time, the American battalion shelled the German positions to the east, over the Second Platoon's camp. Evidence suggests the American artillery had established itself too close to the field hospital. Thus, the Second Platoon became an unintentional target for the Germans.

The day after the attack, while delivering rations to the other platoons, Capt. Joseph Shoham came upon a destroyed 105mm German gun. It was on Elsenborn Ridge, east of the village, near the Siegfried Line. An American military policeman standing next to it pointed out that it was one of the guns that had fired on a field hospital the previous night and that it had been destroyed by counter battery fire.

"I know," said Shoham. "I was there."

To THIS DAY there is no universally agreed-upon explanation as to why the Waffen-SS killed 642 people in Oradour-sur-Glane on the same afternoon that Frances Slanger and the Forty-fifth Field Hospital splashed ashore at Normandy. Some believe the village was massacred in retaliation for the French Resistance's murder of Helmut Kämpfe, a German officer and close friend of Adolf Diekmann, commander of the detachment that committed the atrocity. Others believe the Germans confused Oradour-sur-Glane with Oradour-sur-Vayres, a well-known center of Resistance activity twenty miles away.

Twenty-one soldiers were tried by the French courts in 1953 for their part in the massacre. In the end, two of the defendants were sentenced to death, the rest to prison for between eight to twelve years. The two sentenced to death had their sentences commuted to life. The rest were released long before their sentences were completed.

Three years to the day after the massacre, construction began on an entirely new village. It was completed six years later. The original village has been left as a monument to those who died on June 10, 1944.

• • •

WHEN LØDZ, Poland became the first Jewish ghetto to be sealed by the Germans in April 1940, it was home to 170,000 Jews. On January 19, 1945, when Russian troops liberated the ghetto, only 877 were found alive.

After the war, most of the Jews still alive in Lødz left Poland for Israel, Frances's cousin, Franje, among them. In Lødz today, only a few hundred Jews remain. The city's phone book lists nobody with the name of "Slanger" or "Schlanger."

DESPITE DEADLY new weapons, American battle death rates in World War II shrunk by about half compared to World War I. That was due, in part, to new medicine, such as penicillin, that prevented infection; better doctors, nurses, and medical techniques; and mobile surgical units that stayed close to the action and thus could operate on soldiers much sooner than surgeons could in World War I.

If the army's overall death rate in World War I had continued in World War II, half a million more Americans would not have returned home. The greatest legacy of medical outfits such as the Forty-fifth Field Hospital, then, was the lives they saved—the number of daughters and sons who were born and raised because medics, doctors, and nurses wouldn't let their fathers die.

"If the Forty-fifth couldn't save a man," said Shoham, "he couldn't be saved."

OF ALL THE U.S. women's components in World War II, the Army Nurse Corps sustained the heaviest casualties. Seventeen American nurses were killed in combat in all theaters of operation during World War II. Nearly 18,000 nurses served in Europe. Frances was the lone Army Nurse Corps nurse who landed at Normandy to later die in combat.

The Forty-fifth Field Hospital was disbanded on October 11, 1945, and, unlike many units, never held a reunion. By February 2004, only four of the eighteen nurses who waded ashore on Utah Beach on June 10, 1944, were known to be alive: Sallylou Cummings, Mae Montague, Betty Belanger, and Dottie Richter. Frances Slanger's three Second Platoon tent mates are deceased. Christine Cox, forty-seven, died in 1968 of cardiovascular failure in Burlington, Vermont. Elizabeth Powers, seventy-five, died in 1985 from injuries suffered in a fall in West Roxbury, Massachusetts. Margaret Bowler, eighty-five, died in 1995, of Alzheimer's disease in Millbrae, California.

John Bonzer and Sallylou Cummings, lovers overseas, went their separate ways after the war, she to Wisconsin, he to New Jersey. Neither returned to their "promised ones." But, over time, they found their ways back to each other. They were married August 16, 1948, in Janesville, Wisconsin, and celebrated their fifty-fifth wedding anniversary in August 2003. The same year they were married, *The Saturday Evening Post* magazine published a seven-page, seven-photo feature on Sallylou to show life as a typical nurse. Her movie-star smile was as sweet as ever. The Bonzers, both eighty-four, live in Eugene, Oregon, where, before retiring, John worked as a doctor and Sallylou as a nurse. They raised four children.

Among others from the Forty-fifth Field Hospital, Joseph Shoham, who recovered completely from his wounded arm, spent fifty-eight years as a dentist in Long Island and Latham, New York. He retired, at age eighty-six, in the spring of 2000 and later moved to Reston, Virginia, to be near a son. He and the young woman he eloped with in the Bronx, Ethel, celebrated their sixty-fourth wedding anniversary in December 2003. They have two sons. Shoham still collects not only beetles, but butterflies, dental instruments, and odd-shaped teeth.

Capt. Fred Michalove, the softhearted man who'd been

given the farm-fresh egg by Frances, sold advertising for, and began his own, trade magazines in the years after the war. He and his wife, Helen, had two sons. He died August 27, 2002, two days after his ninetieth birthday.

After the war, Isadore "Tiny" Schwartz returned to Quincy, Massachusetts, where he served as senior surgeon at Quincy Hospital for more than thirty-five years and as chief of surgery at Jewish Memorial Hospital in Boston. His first wife, with whom he had a son and a daughter, died in 1971 and he remarried. Over the years, Schwartz occasionally visited Eva Slanger in nearby Roxbury. "Whenever Frances's name was mentioned," one of her nephews, Jerry Sidman, said, "his eyes would automatically tear up—just like that." In 1994, Schwartz died of a heart attack in Sarasota, Florida, just short of fifty years since the night Frances Slanger died in his arms.

EVA SLANGER never completely recovered from losing David and Frances within thirty months of each other. She was plagued by diabetes and heart problems during the 1950s, but she lived with, and remained close to, her remaining family. She was happiest in the kitchen, especially making meals for other people. And she rarely passed up an opportunity to talk to visitors about her daughter the war hero. She put together a small memorial in the living room with pictures and mementos of Frances.

Eva lived with her daughter, Sally, and her family in Hull, Massachusetts, until her death on November 23, 1957, following a heart attack. She was seventy-five. Frances's sister, Sally, died in 1997 at age ninety-one, leaving three sons:

Irwin Sidman, at sixty-five the eldest of Frances's nephews, was seven years old when Frances had hugged him good-bye in Hull, Massachusetts, and headed for Fort Devens. He is a travel agent in Boston.

Jerry Sidman was three years old when Frances left for the army. Now sixty-one, he lives in Attleboro, Massachusetts. He is retired from the warehouse business.

Francis Slanger Sidman, fifty-eight, is the youngest of Frances's nephews. Sally was pregnant with him the day the telegram arrived with news about her sister's death. Born June 17, 1945, two weeks before the *Frances Y. Slanger* was launched, he was named in honor of his aunt. He lives in Lakeland, Florida, where a menorah made from the shell fired during Frances's burial service in Boston sits on a shelf. After years of moving from job to job, he believes he's finally found his calling, one that his mother always told him he was destined to find.

He is a nurse.

AFTERWORD

In September 2001, I flew to Europe to follow the trail of Frances Slanger. On my first full day in France, I viewed the chillingly well-preserved remains of Oradour-sur-Glane. It was here on June 10, 1944—at the precise hour Frances and the Forty-fifth Field Hospital nurses waded ashore at Utah Beach—that German soldiers massacred 642 men, women, and children.

It is one thing to read a description of an atrocity; it is quite another to see the crumbled village that a few hours of fiery horror left behind. I saw scorched watches that never again marked time, sewing machines that never again made dresses, and dolls that never again were cradled in little girls' arms.

"Man's inhumanity to man," a Frenchman muttered as we left the village.

Later that day, my wife, Sally, and I drove to Normandy on a route similar to the one taken by the German troops after the attack. The beauty of the French countryside numbed the pain we'd felt while viewing the remains of Oradour-sur-Glane. At dusk, we arrived on the Normandy coast and found an ocean-front hotel in the little town of Grandcamp-Maisy, midway between Omaha Beach and Utah Beach. I popped open our room's window and watched gentle waves lap ashore.

The Normandy coast was beautiful and benign. When we'd first seen Omaha Beach, a couple of sand yachts slalomed beside surf once colored red with the blood of American soldiers. A miniature golf course perched above a beach once strewn with bodies. The Utah Beach Internet Café welcomed customers along dunes once littered with German hedgehogs.

Given such surroundings, it was hard to imagine the bloody carnage of D-Day and the brutal fighting in Normandy that followed. All of which made me wonder about the relevance of a book about a World War II nurse who had died nearly six decades ago. Hadn't we, after all, left such atrocities to the history books?

The answer came at dinner. We were awaiting our order when a man from Dublin, Ireland, at the next table said, "Excuse me, but are you Americans?"

"We are," I said.

"Have you heard?"

"Heard what?"

"Terrorists have blown up the World Trade Center," he said. "And the Pentagon. Just hours ago."

The news on this eleventh day of September 2001 was so horrific I momentarily thought the man was kidding or drunk or both. Later, I experienced an eerie juxtaposition of time, place, and history: listening to the sound of the Normandy surf while viewing CNN images of the collapsing World Trade Center.

Evil, I was reminded, never goes away. It simply lurks in the shadows of time, morphs to fit the technological advances, and springs on another generation. Hitler, bin Laden, Saddam Hussein—the monsters change, the methods change, but the motivating madness does not. My hearing the news of devastation in my homeland was no different from a citizen of Oradour-sur-Glane visiting Limoges for a day in 1944—and later hearing of the Germans' attack on his hometown. In both cases, evil unexpectedly exploded on the innocent.

Though we'd rather not believe it, bullies prowl the world. And to stop those bullies, lives must sometimes be sacrificed. Thus do I believe the Frances Slanger story is as relevant now as it was then.

At Oradour-sur-Glane, there's but one word on the gate

entering the "martyred village": *Remember.* It is the inspiration behind other places I visited such as Utah Beach and its memorial, the U.S. Holocaust Memorial Museum in Washington, D.C., and the cemetery above Omaha Beach. We must remember the atrocities of the past to prevent such atrocities in the future.

Still, we're remiss if we don't also remember those, such as Frances, who dared, if even in seemingly small ways, to resist such evil. "I think of Frances as something of a 'reformer,'" Capt. Joseph Shoham once told me in his Latham, New York, living room. "She took something and improved on it. You go through your life thinking: 'What could I have done?' She *did* it. She left the world better than she found it."

Others, such as Adolf Hitler, do just the opposite. But then, it's tempting to shoulder a Hitler or bin Laden with the label of "evil" and validate the rest of the world as "good." It isn't that simple. "The essence of tragedy," wrote I. F. Stone in *The Nation* the same month the Forty-fifth Field Hospital Unit landed in Normandy, "is not the doing of evil by evil men but the doing of evil by good men, out of weakness, indecision, sloth, inability to act in accordance with what they know to be right."

Aleksandr Solzhenitsyn, the Nobel Prize–winning Russian novelist who spent eight years in prison and labor camps before being exiled from the then–Soviet Union, put it well in his book, *The Gulag Archipelago:* "The line separating good and evil passes not through states, not between classes, nor between political parties either, but right through every human heart."

In my nearly three years of researching and writing *American Nightingale*, I made numerous trips to the house of Sallylou Cummings Bonzer, who lives only ten minutes from me. At times, I'd find this eighty-four year-old woman on her hands and knees, toiling since sunup in her garden, wearing the same field jacket she wore in France. And I came to realize that few, if any, of the people who drove past her day in and day out—her own neighbors—knew that this remarkable woman once slept in foxholes, ate K-rations, and eased the fears of critically wounded soldiers, all to help Allied forces return freedom to the world.

The World War II generation has never been a perfect generation, but I believe it has been a noble generation. A generation that resisted evil through great sacrifice. And yet has rarely sought the limelight that it is due. In some cases, I interviewed adult children of nurses and doctors from the Forty-fifth who had no idea of the heroics their parents had performed. For whatever reason—mainly, I presume, modesty and the pain of looking back—their mothers and fathers had never told them.

"We just did what needed to be done," the late Capt. Fred Michalove told me from his assisted-living home in Rhode Island.

Now, this generation is leaving us. Of a fighting force of twelve million, more than a thousand WWII veterans are dying every day. One Forty-fifth nurse, 2d Lt. Margaret Fielden, died even as I was trying to find her. Michalove died shortly after I interviewed him. Joseph Shoham once included a poignant "P.S." in a letter he sent me. "In the event yours truly is no longer on this planet when the book comes out," he wrote in chicken-scratch, "would you please see that my sons receive copies."

He and the others seem to take a quiet pride in what they did, not that the ghosts haven't lingered. Nurse Betty Belanger had nightmares for years after the war, most of them the same: German soldiers coming to get her. When Michalove was telling me about coming ashore at Utah Beach, he repeatedly stopped and took me back to England, as if it were too painful to come ashore and see the dangling paratroopers. And nearly six decades after it happened, he could not tell the story of Frances giving him the farm-fresh egg—he told it three times—without crying.

This is a generation whose legacy is a deep sense of purpose, a quiet sense of pride, and an indefatigable sense of sacrifice. Their best war memories are simple: each other. Some met spouses during the war, people they've been with for more than half a century. John and Sallylou Bonzer still talk occasionally to Joseph Shoham even though they live on opposite sides of the country and haven't seen each other since 1945.

In Dover, Delaware, as Mae "Monty" Montague was moving to smaller quarters, a daughter recommended throwing out a painting of a cobblestone street in England, flanked by houses. "No, no, no," protested Monty. "That's the painting that reminds me of your father and I walking to see Frances Slanger."

When I visited Montague months later, there was the painting, hanging proudly on her apartment wall.

AFTER IMMERSING myself so deeply in the life of Frances Slanger, the place where she died in Belgium had taken on a nearly mythical image in my mind. But when I got there, I found it to be a simple country village.

I stood in the field where the Second Platoon had pitched its tents and where Frances had written her letter. As in Normandy, it was hard to imagine death in such a pastoral scene. A cow mooed in the distance. A light rain pattered on the country road. Birds flitted about. I walked around a bit, scanned the countryside, and tried to imagine Frances writing to *Stars and Stripes* in a tent, by flashlight, on that rainy October night in 1944.

I gathered a handful of small stones for her nephews—to go with the sand I'd gathered at Utah Beach for the Forty-fifth nurses and doctors back home. I took a few photographs, walked back to my rental car, then left. There was one final stop I needed to make in following the journey of Frances Slanger: the American Cemetery and Memorial at Henri-Chapelle. It is here where Frances was first laid to rest.

Sally and I arrived on a drizzly Saturday morning, a nearly colorless day save for the blur of bicyclists who raced past the cemetery entrance. Some 50,000 people visit the cemetery each year, including a few thousand Americans, but on this day we essentially had the place to ourselves, except for Caroline Oliver, a guide who spoke far better English than we spoke French or German.

From a terrace overlooking the cemetery, the white marble crosses and occasional Stars of David stretched out seemingly forever across the carpet of green. The rows were so straight— the eight-section symmetry so neat and tidy—that, from above, it all looked as innocent as a fabric pattern. But here lay 7,989 American soldiers, most killed in the Battle of the Bulge, the Battle for Aachen, and the Battle of the Hürtgen Forest. We walked along a wall that honors 450 soldiers whose bodies were never found. An American flag fluttered lightly at half-staff, a handful of bouquets having been placed at its base in remembrance of those who had died four days before in the terrorist attacks back home.

Later, with Oliver, we talked about Frances, the cemetery, and the type of people who come to visit the cemetery. "One day a soldier was here whose job, back then, was to bury the dead," said Oliver. "He told me you could see the fear, the agony, the horror on their faces."

The image only solidified the sense of hopelessness this cemetery experience was instilling in me. The headstones were reminders of a time when the world was sick; now, the half-staffed flag was a reminder that we'd had a tragic relapse. From Normandy to here, we had seen far too many world war memorials and far too many photographs in French newspapers of the crumbled World Trade Center. The rain was falling harder. My spirits were sagging. It was time to go home.

We were gathering our belongings in Oliver's office when an older man of World War II vintage poked his head in the doorway. He held a bouquet of daisies in his hand. He was German. He spoke only broken English and, I realized, was seeking a vase.

"What soldier are the flowers for?" asked Oliver.

At first, the man did not understand, but when Oliver asked him again in German, he did. His answer, in broken English, brought to mind fires burning low and soldiers—perhaps the world itself—being nursed back from the dying embers, as was done all the time in field hospitals across the ETO, according to Frances Slanger.

"For New York," he said. "And Washington."

Portions of letters written to Stars and Stripes *after Frances Slanger's editorial had been published and before soldiers realized she had died:*

"You will probably receive many, many letters relative to your article in S&S. There will be many lads up front who will have time only to read your message while on the 'go,' murmur an inaudible 'God bless her,' and crawl on their way without having even a chance to sit in a tent and by candlelight scrawl a line your way as I'm doing now.

"Your article was a real example of the sincere great heartedness which is an intangible tie between us as soldiers and Americans."

—Staff Sgt. Jim Squires, November 8, 1944

"The determination and will of the army nurses shall never be surpassed—not even by the GI himself."

—Warrant Officer Russell Preston, November 8, 1944

". . . Reliving the suffering. Cleaning up the blood, guts, and filth of us from the battlefields. Dying with us. Dreaming and sweating out the time with us. . . . Oh, you know what I want to say. God bless every one of them. These influences will always be with us."

—Sgt. John W. O'Donnell, November 8, 1944

"Orchids to them all. After I was knocked out it was a nurse who set the flame going to the little spark that was left in me. It's about time someone did give them some credit."

—Pvt. Alfred Garraffa

"I haven't heard the 'hi ya, babe" from a wounded Yank, but I have seen the look in their eyes which says, 'here is a real American girl who has given up the finer things in life back home to help us over here.' I have seen these nurses work till they could drop—working to kindle that fire again in some 'Joe' who had done his part. They don't all get Bronze Stars though God knows they deserve them. But I'm sure there is a bigger and better star shining somewhere for them."

—T/4 Harry Bachiochi, November 8, 1944

Portions of letters written to Stars and Stripes *after soldiers realized Frances Slanger had died:*

"With tear-dimmed eyes, I read your announcement that [Frances] was killed that very night, immediately after mailing her heartfelt message to you. An inner conscience keeps asking . . . why? Why did this kind, noble soul have to die? And like always a feeling of futility overwhelms us. However, we know that Frances Slanger did not die in vain. The spirit of mercy, goodness and everything fine that was in her—and all those mud-grimed GIs she loved so tenderly—will live forever in the hearts of decent men and women everywhere. . . ."

—*Edward Kohn, November 24, 1944*

"I cannot say how much I was moved by this bad news—as were all GIs. Thoughts occurred that 'S&S' might be helpful in materializing a memorial for her—a statue, a park, a hospital. . . .

"But more than that, it is rather for us to be dedicated to the task before us: Killing the German savages who, thru fascism, brought war to the world—killing women and children, torturing whole peoples, attempting to extinguish culture, civilization itself.

"We in Belgium, and others in France, Holland and now Germany, may never be present at any memorial service for this heroine, but her parents may be assured that we all mourn with them and pledge to fight harder so that the world may forever be rid of the cause of her death."

—*Pvt. Leon Straus, Headquarters battery,*
559th Field Artillery Battalion

"We request a reprint of Lt. Slanger's grand epistle. We all feel it worth repeating."

—*117th Infantry Regiment, 30th Infantry Division,*
November 25, 1944

"To me, Frances will be an idol, a living symbol of Americanism, a true picture of those things for which we are fighting. Her life and her death are, in themselves, beautiful. Beautiful because she used them as she wanted and as God would want: dedicated to serving, comforting, and healing.

"Lincoln said—'Who gave their lives that others might live.' So true is this of Frances and so true is it of the hundreds of girls who would, and are, doing the same thing, the hundreds of other girls who have come all that way with us, making the same sacrifices, living under the same conditions and ducking the same bullets.

"Our sorrow can never be appropriately expressed; we just hope that Frances can somehow know the way we feel about her and how much she and those like her meant to us."

—*William R. Phillips, 118th Infantry, November 23, 1944*

"Men, we owe these nurses the highest debt of appreciation and the utmost respect. . . . They have proved, beyond doubt, that they have the 'guts' of the best soldier.

"All praise, all honor and all respect we shower on the Army Nurse Corps cannot begin to compare to the glory each of them earns each day as true American Soldiers."

—*Lt. Chester S. Wright Jr., November 24, 1944*

"We think she should be awarded the Congressional Medal of Honor and also be placed in the Hall of Fame in Washington, D.C. Gallant Heroines and Heroes always die a gallant death."

—*Pvt. Jack Hoss and three signers, no date*

"Miss Slanger shall never be forgotten by thousands of GIs, particularly those who she must have so patiently and efficiently served. The tribute required would be beyond the scope of mere words. We are certain that every man in the service feels the same way. We regret exceedingly that Frances Slanger could not know of our sentiments before her passing. Here's for a great person from a great nation and one less question of doubt as to 'Why We Are Fighting.' "

—*Technician Fourth Class Ed A. Ferris, no date*

"[These nurses] will stay by your Bud when everyone else says it's 'only time.' A man is supposed to be a mature person. But after seeing those frail nurses it makes you soft. I read the first letter Lt. Slanger wrote and it touched me. . . . After reading [in] the paper of her misfortune, I wanted to cry. Nothing never means much to me. It takes people like her to change Joes like me.

"I hope you can read this. I know it is not the best. But it is the way millions feel."

—*Name obscured, no date*

"Her letter was enough to make a guy hold up his head, throw out his chest and step out with more pride and confidence than he ever had before."

—*Staff Sgt. Jo Chasin, November 23, 1944*

"Dear Mom [Eva Slanger]: Please pardon my lack of good manners in addressing you as Mom but having served as a brother in arms with our Frances I feel more or less entitled to the privilege so 'Mom' it is.

"Having myself been under shell fire on numerous occasions, I can speak with authority on the inward feelings one has during a barrage and hope you find some comfort in my statement when I say the fear encountered is not as much for one's own personal safety as it is for the grief and inconvenience an accident would cause to those loved ones left behind.

"Frances was no different in this respect, as her comrades

said her main concern was the grief she was causing you. . . . It is just one of the damnable effects of war and only proves that they also serve who wait at home.

"I could very easily write that you should be brave and accept fate in [realizing] that Frances died a heroine's death, but being the father of a small son and daughter, know my words would be useless as it all goes much deeper than that.

"If I were in your place I know that I would remember Frances from the time of her first cry to the last parting when she sailed away from you forever.

"Yes, all those little things she ever did will be vividly recalled to you so many times during the day, her first tooth, her first step, her first pigtails, her first beau, her first party dress, and all those other things that go with raising a daughter.

"You must have been very proud of her when she first donned the uniform of the Army Nurse Corps and what a real soldier she was. You have a right to be proud of her as she lived and died [an] ideal—to aid and comfort her fellow man.

"In closing I might add that if fate ever deems it necessary that I should spend time in a convalescent hospital, that hospital will bear the name Frances Slanger. As for you, Mom, the greatest memorial your Frances will ever have is that little part of every GI Joe's heart that is especially reserved for Frances and the girls in the Army Nurse Corps.

"May God ease your pain in this hour of need and convince you that our girl has not died in vain."

—*Lt. Raymond E. Sanders, November 26, 1944*

"If it is humanly possible to preserve her memory we suggest naming a hospital ship in her honor so when this terrible Holocaust is over we can carry her ideals into a world of peace."

—*Pvt. B. Mallott and five cosigners, November 25, 1944*

SOURCE NOTES

CHAPTER 1

All chapter quotations are from Frances Slanger's chapbook, found in the Frances Slanger Collection, History of Nursing Archives, The Howard Gotlieb Archival Research Center at Boston University.

Many details of the voyage of the USS *William N. Pendleton* were found in the report of the "Office of the Chief of Surgical Services, 128th Evacuation Hospital, APO 230," in the National Archives II, College Park, Md. (Nurses from the 128th Evac were on the ship along with those from the Forty-fifth Field Hospital.)

Forty-fifth Field Hospital nurses Sallylou Cummings, Betty Belanger, Dottie Richter, and Mae Montague offered firsthand accounts of the voyage.

Physical details of the *Pendleton* were obtained from the American Merchant Marine Museum, Kings Point, N.Y. The Steamship Historical Society of America, Baltimore, Md., provided a photograph of the ship. Another invaluable source was Peter Elphick's *Liberty: The Ships That Won the War* (Annapolis, Maryland: Naval Institute Press, 2001).

Frances Slanger's "Buddy Book," found in The Howard Gotlieb Archival Research Center, provided wide, if not deep, insight into Frances. As Frances left Fort Devens in Massachusetts, Fort Rucker in Alabama, and Camp Gordon in Georgia, fellow soldiers made good-bye comments about her that proved extremely helpful.

Her chapbook, also found in Boston University's archives, includes a wealth of information. The book contains dozens of poems and stories she wrote and inspirational nuggets from other writing she admired. For example, the chapbook included the newsletter from her father's lodge about dropping "a pebble in the water. . . ." Other poems by Frances were found at the National Museum of American Jewish Military History in Washington, D.C.

A copy of Frances's record of service, showing the specific stints she spent at four training camps, was found in The Howard Gotlieb Archival Research Center. However, her official military records—and those of the rest of the Forty-fifth's individuals—were lost in a 1973 fire at the National Personnel Records Center in St. Louis.

Information on Dawid Schlanger's immigration to America was gleaned from U.S. Department of Labor Naturalization Service records at U.S. District Court, Boston, Massachusetts. The records showed that Dawid lived with his cousin, Jacob Grossman, when he first arrived, and was a fruit peddler.

Genealogical experts Shirley Rotbein Flaum of Houston, Texas, and Petje Schröder, of Lødz, Poland, traced the Schlanger family tree.

The unpublished personal memoirs of Sara Brenner, written in 1981, provided insightful details of life in Poland around the turn of the century.

Frances Slanger's date of birth is debatable. However, the preponderance of evidence suggests August 13, 1913, the date I've used, is accurate. Some school records indicate she was born July 8, 1914. And the headstone on her grave notes she was age thirty when she died, which would square with a birth in July 1914. However, genealogical records from Lødz, her father's Petition for Naturalization papers, the *Nieuw Amsterdam*'s manifest, and military records all show her birth date as August 13, 1913, meaning she most likely died at age thirty-one.

A number of books offered the social and political nuances of Lødz soon after the turn of the century, foremost among them: Chava Rosenfarb's *Of Lødz and Love* (Syracuse, N.Y.: Syracuse University Press, 2000); I. J. Singer's *The Brothers Ashkenazi* (London: Allison & Busby, 1980); William Glickman's *In the Mirror of Literature: The Economic Life of the Jews in Poland as Reflected in*

Yiddish Literature, 1914–1939 (New York: Living Books, Inc., 1966); Celia Heller's *On the Edge of Destruction* (New York: Columbia University Press, 1977); and Joseph Marcus's *Social and Political History of the Jews in Poland, 1919–1939* (Berlin: Mouton Publishers, 1983).

An insightful overview of the Battle of Łódz was gleaned from Girard Lindsley McEntee's *Military History of the World War* (New York: Charles Scribner's Sons, 1937). The soldier's-eye view was dramatically captured by *The Times* (London), December 7, 1914, and January 22, 1915.

CHAPTER 2

Some of the physical details of Oradour-sur-Glane were gleaned from a personal visit to the French village, which has been left as a memorial for those who died. But the specifics of what transpired in the horrific hours of June 10, 1944, including Albert Roumbi's hopes of proposing to his sweetheart, were taken from eyewitness accounts shared by survivors and reported in the following excellent books: *War for An Afternoon* by Jens Kause (New York: Random House, 1968); *Martyred Village* by Sarah Framer (Berkeley, California: University of California Press, 1999); and *Oradour-sur-Glane: A Vision of Horror* by Guy Pauchou and Pierre Masfrand (The National Association of the Families of the Martyrs of Oradour-sur-Glane, 1997). In addition, I'm indebted to the website of Mike Williams (www.oradour.btinternet.co.uk/).

In an interview, a cousin of Slanger's, Sylvia Fine of Lakehurst, N.J., told me of Frances being detained at Ellis Island because of the eye infection. Immigration records confirmed this.

The American Family Immigration History Center website (www.ellisislandrecords.org) provided a copy of the manifest of the *Nieuw Amsterdam*, which confirmed the September 7, 1920, arrival of Regina, Chaja, and Freidel Slanger. It also provided information on the number, names, and countries represented of those on board, along with a photograph and general facts of the ship.

Details of what the three would have experienced while pass-

ing through Ellis Island in 1920 were obtained by personally visit-
ing the island and from a number of enlightening books, including:
Bertha Boody's *A Psychological Study of Immigrant Children at Ellis
Island* (Baltimore: The Williams & Wilkins Company, 1926); Ann
Novotny's *Strangers at the Door* (New York: Bantam Books, 1972);
Thomas M. Pitkin's *Keepers of the Gate: A History of Ellis Island* (New
York: New York University Press, 1975); William Carlson Smith's
*Americans in the Making: The Natural History of the Assimilation of
Immigrants* (New York: D. Appleton-Century Company, 1939); and
Island of Hope, Island of Tears by David M. Brownstone, Douglass L.
Brownstone, and Irene M. Franck (New York: Rawson, Wade
Publishers, Inc., 1979).

Frances Slanger's struggle to get ashore at Utah Beach was
witnessed by Sallylou Cummings and well-documented in newspaper articles.

CHAPTER 3

I was able to re-create the Forty-fifth's landing at Normandy
through eyewitness accounts of four nurses—Cummings,
Montague, Richter, and Belanger—and from Capt. Fred
Michalove, Capt. Joseph Shoham, Capt. John Bonzer, and Pvt.
William King, whose landing craft hit the beach shortly after the
nurses arrived. A report, "Office of the Chief of Surgical Services,
128th Evacuation Hospital, APO 230," found in the National
Archives, added precise details in terms of timing and enemy fire.
The Forty-fifth Field Hospital's Company Morning Reports also
provided useful information—for example, a confirmation of doc-
tors and nurses who remember a dental officer, Capt. Emanuel D.
Berson, being wounded at Utah Beach. In an interview, Berson personally confirmed the wounding.

In addition, a number of books added detail, among the best,
Jonathan Gawne's *Spearheading D-Day* (Paris: Histoire &
Collections, 1999); *D-Day: Operation Overlord*, edited by Tony Hall
(New York: Smithmark Publishers Inc., 1993); Stephen E.
Ambrose's *D-Day* (New York: Touchstone, 1994); and Cornelius

Ryan's *The Longest Day* (New York: Simon and Schuster, Inc., 1959).

Nobody did more to help me understand life in Boston's South End in the 1920s and 1930s than Milton Zola, who grew up three blocks away from Frances Slanger and knew her. Not only did Zola provide memories of Frances, her father, and the South End, but he secured a map so detailed it actually listed owners of individual properties—and he took me on a personal tour of the area. Joseph Yanoff, whose family was close to the Slangers and lived just down the street, also offered details.

The noted historian Theodore H. White, two years younger than Frances Slanger, grew up only a few miles south of her and wrote eloquently of that time and place in his book, *In Search of History: A Personal Adventure* (New York: Warner Books, 1978). Among other books with helpful information were *The Jews of Boston* by Jonathan D. Sarna and Ellen Smith (Boston: The Combined Jewish Philanthropies of Greater Boston, Inc., 1995) and *The Great Interlude: Neglected Events and Persons from the First World War to the Depression* by Francis Russell (New York: McGraw-Hill Book Company, 1964).

In addition, the Boston Public Library provided a number of photographs of the South End and Roxbury areas during that time, showing, for example, what the Dudley Street Terminal looked like. A Boston City Directory confirmed where the family lived since Dawid Schlanger's arrival in 1913.

Frances's rooftop "hideaway," her dog "Yip-Yip," and her pet parakeet were prominent in a personal photo album passed on to her three nephews, Irwin Sidman, Jerry Sidman, and Francis Sidman.

Her chapbook included photographs of Frances and classmates at Abraham Lincoln Intermediate School and at the High School of Practical Arts, school papers, and comments from teachers on those school papers.

An extremely helpful book on understanding the assimilation of Jewish women was *American Jewish History*, particularly Volume 3, edited by Jeffrey S. Gurock: *East European Jews in America, 1880–1920: Immigration and Adaption* (New York: Routledge, 1998).

Among others: Rose Cohen's *Out of the Shadow* (Ithaca, N.Y.: Cornell University Press, 1995); *Lives and Voices: A Collection of American Jewish Memoirs*, edited by Stanley F. Chyet (Philadelphia: The Jewish Publication Society of America, 1972); Kathie Friedman-Kasaba's *Memories of Migration: Gender, Ethnicity, and Work in the Lives of Jewish and Italian Women in New York, 1870–1924* (Albany, N.Y.: State University of New York Press, 1996); *The Jewish Woman in America*, by Charlotte Baum, Paula Hyman, and Sonya Michel (New York: Plume, 1975); *Jewish Women in America: An Historical Encyclopedia*, edited by Paul E. Hyman and Deborah Dash Moore (New York: American Jewish Historical Society, 1998); and S. J. Kleinberg's *Women in the United States, 1830–1945* (New Brunswick, N.J.: Rutgers University Press, 1999).

Throughout the book, Boston newspapers—the *Globe, Record-Advertiser, Traveler,* and *Herald*—were used to determine weather conditions on particular days.

CHAPTER 4

Frances Slanger's passion to be a nurse was well expressed by her in a letter she wrote to Boston City Hospital's School of Nursing, found in the Frances Slanger Collection, History of Nursing Archives, The Howard Gotlieb Archival Research Center at Boston University. The same letter detailed her going to the School of Nursing and later to the Children's Hospital in Wellesley Hills, seeking advice on how she might become a nurse. In addition, Slanger family friend Joseph Yanoff provided insight into Frances's nursing inclinations in how she helped take care of his two disabled brothers.

The best general information I gathered on Jewish women and nursing was from Evelyn Benson's excellent book, *As We See Ourselves* (Indianapolis, Indiana: Sigma Theta Tau International Honor Society of Nursing, 2001).

The Forty-second Field Hospital's Annual Report, found at the National Archives, shows how overwhelmed doctors and nurses were on their first night ashore. (The Forty-fifth's nurses were supporting the Forty-second's doctors, whose nurses hadn't yet arrived on June

10, 1944.) Among other details, the report revealed the incredible fact that "17 truckloads of wounded waited admittance."

In addition, the "Third Auxiliary Team History APO 230," also found at National Archives, provided further details about what the Forty-fifth's nurses experienced that first night. (Surgeons from the Third Auxiliary Unit were part of that June 10–11, 1944, hybrid team that included the Forty-fifth's nurses.)

For a better understanding of war in the ETO through the eyes of the men who fought it, I relied heavily on Gerald F. Linderman's *The World Within War* (New York: The Free Press, 1997) and Stephen E. Ambrose's *Citizen Soldiers* (New York: Touchstone, 1997). Two compilations of stories from American journalists who witnessed war in the ETO provided not only great background information but literary inspiration: *Reporting World War II: American Journalism 1938–1946* (New York: The Library of America, 1995) and *Reporting World War II: Part Two, American Journalism 1944–1946* (New York: The Library of America, 1995). Nothing I read about nurses in Europe was as powerful as a piece in the latter book called "U.S.A. Tent Hospital," by Lee Miller, one of many female World War II correspondents—and also a noted *Life* magazine photographer.

Photos from dozens of books helped put war in perspective. But I found that paintings, sketches, and drawings by combat artists brought home the horrors of battle to an even deeper level. The finest book with such visual recollections is *They Drew Fire: Combat Artists of World War II*, edited by Brian Lanker and Nicole Newnham (New York: TV Books, 2000). Also helpful was James Jones's *WWII* (New York: Ballantine Books, 1975).

In addition, I relied heavily on photos taken by members of the Forty-fifth, including Cummings, Bonzer, Richter, Shoham, and Belanger.

CHAPTER 5

Joseph Shoham, even at age eighty-seven, boasts a stellar memory and provided considerable insight into Frances Slanger and the

Second Platoon. Much of the anecdotal details I used were mined from the former army cook/dentist/chronicler. He kept a journal of each place the Forty-fifth moved on a particular date. And spoke, with great pride, about his beetle collecting.

Other insight on the Forty-fifth's advance across France and Belgium came from Michalove, Bonzer, Pvt. William King, and Sgt. Charles Willen. Cummings, Belanger, Richter, and Montague offered details on nursing life.

The initial part of this chapter, detailed by Shoham, was made more vivid by an Associated Press photograph taken of Frances combing her hair while sitting on an overturned wash basin. It appeared in a number of U.S. papers.

Information on the High School of Practical Arts was gleaned from a 1925 brochure on the school and from stories in the school's literary magazine, *The Shuttle*, for which Frances wrote. Frances's increasing absences and slipping grades during the Depression were well documented in her school records, filed at the Boston School District archives. The same records also included information on her job at Massachusetts Knitting Mills, including her $13-a-week pay.

Specific information on David Slanger's health came from the Massachusetts State Department of Health, Registrar of Vital Records, Dorchester, Massachusetts. That Frances struggled to get through nursing school was clearly evident in her records, which were found amid files on Boston City Hospital's School of Nursing in the History of Nursing Archives at Boston University. Additional insight was offered by one of Frances's classmates, Hazelle Ferguson, among the first black nurses to break Boston City's quotas for African-American women.

Frances's loathing of overbearing supervisors was the theme of an article she wrote and had published in the September 1940 issue of the *American Journal of Nursing*. Her personal photo album includes a picture of her rocking a black baby on the roof of the hospital. Her oldest nephew, Irwin Sidman, retold the story of Frances returning to the Slanger/Sidman home in emotional turmoil after having been reprimanded by a supervisor for spending too much time with children on her ward.

The German zeppelin floating over Roxbury—and the reaction of young Jewish people—was documented by Theodore H. White in his previously noted book, *In Search of History: A Personal Adventure.*

To understand the Lødz Ghetto during World War II, I relied heavily on *Poland's Ghettos at War* by Alfred Katz (New York: Twayne Publishers, Inc., 1970). However, the actual journals written by Jews living in the ghetto proved even more enlightening. Particularly insightful and gritty were *The Diary of Dawid Sierakowiak: Five Notebooks from the Lodz Ghetto* (New York: Oxford University Press, 1996); *Lodz Ghetto*, edited by Alan Adelson and Robert Lapides (New York: Viking, 1989); and *The Chronicle of the Lodz Ghetto 1941–1944*, edited by Lucjan Dobrosyzycki (Yale, Conn.: Yale University Press, 1984).

America's response to the Jews' plight during World War II is well documented in Arthur D. Morse's *While Six Million Died* (New York: Random House, 1967) and David S. Wyman's *The Abandonment of the Jews: America and the Holocaust, 1941–1945* (New York: The New Press, 1984).

CHAPTER 6

Beyond the eyewitnesses of those in the Forty-fifth, the day-to-day life of army nurses was detailed by a number of sources. At Schlesinger Library at the Radcliffe Institute for Advanced Study, at Harvard University in Cambridge, Massachusetts, the papers of Associated Press reporter Ruth Cowan contained a number of newspaper stories she wrote on army nurses, including one specifically on the Forty-fifth's Second Platoon.

Books that provided insight on nurses in the ETO were Diane Burke Fessler's *No Time for Fear: Voices of American Military Nurses in World War II* (East Lansing, Mich.: Michigan State University Press, 1996); Betsy Kuhn's *Angels of Mercy: The Army Nurses of World War II* (New York: Atheneum, 1999); and Iris Carpenter's *No Woman's World* (Cambridge: The Riverside Press, 1946).

Elizabeth M. Norman's *We Band of Angels* (New York: Pocket Books, 1999) deals with a different theater of war, the South Pacific, but has no equal among stories of nurses of World War II in terms of its depth and drama.

By far the most insightful magazine article on nurses in the ETO was a piece by Ernest O. Hauser in the *Saturday Evening Post* (March 10, 1945, p. 13).

A number of books provided exhaustive detail about the Army Nurse Corps and its history, including Barbara Brooks Tomblin's *G.I. Nightingales* (Lexington, Kentucky: The University Press of Kentucky, 1996) and Mary T. Sarnecky's exhaustively detailed *A History of the U.S. Army Nurse Corps* (Philadelphia: University of Pennsylvania Press, 1999).

The letter Frances Slanger wrote after the death of the young mother at Boston City Hospital, found in Boston University's Special Collections, provided deep insight into her thoughts on war. Her military motivation as a Jew was detailed by Sylvia Andelman Sokol, first commander of Frances Y. Slanger Post No. 313, in an interview.

The death of the Jewish mother and child was from the diary of Dawid Sierakowiak, found in *Lodz Ghetto* (New York: Viking, 1989), edited by Alan Adelson and Robert Lapides.

I far better understood Frances's struggle of whether to stay with her parents or go off to war after reading Carol S. Pearson's *Awakening the Heroes Within* (San Francisco: HarperSanFrancisco, 1991), which brought to light Frances's caregiver nature.

By far the most comprehensive book in helping me understand the "hows" and "whens" behind the Germans' murder of the Jews was the chillingly honest *The Holocaust Chronicle* (Lincoln, Illinois: Publications International Ltd., 2001).

A number of letters from the Army Nurse Corps, found in the Frances Slanger Collection, History of Nursing Archives, The Howard Gotlieb Archival Research Center at Boston University, offered detailed information about Frances's attempts to become an army nurse.

Irwin Sidman, Frances's oldest nephew, recalled Frances's departure from home for the army.

CHAPTER 7

To understand life in the medical tents of a World War II field hospital in the ETO, I relied on a number of well-written books, foremost among them Albert E. Cowdrey's *Fighting for Life* (New York: The Free Press, 1994). In addition, an article by Stephen E. Ambrose in *American Heritage* magazine (November 1997) was helpful.

I benefited greatly from reading manuals that officers in the ETO were issued, among them: the *Medical Field Manual* (Washington, D.C.: War Department, 1941); *The Officer's Guide* (Harrisburg, Pennsylvania: The Military Service Publishing Co., 1943); *Medical Department Units of a Theater of Operations* (Washington, D.C.: War Department, 1945); *Army Life* (Washington, D.C.: War Department, 1944); and *Medical Soldier's Handbook* (Harrisburg, Pennsylvania: The Military Service Publishing Co., 1942).

The Story of the Medical Service, ETO, a publication overseen by Maj. Gen. Paul Hawley, the U.S. Army's chief surgeon during World War II, explained well the process of treating and evacuating a wounded soldier. It also included an extremely helpful aerial photograph of a field hospital—ironically, the Forty-fifth's Third Platoon.

A collection of poetry written by nurses, *Between the Heartbeats* (Iowa City, Iowa: University of Iowa Press, 1995) helped me better understand the hearts and minds of nurses.

Frances's care of her childhood friend, Milton Zola, at Boston City Hospital in 1941 was recalled by *"Motle"* himself in an interview in Boston.

The little French girl whose parents had been killed by a booby trap was recalled by Capt. Fred Michalove, Pvt. William King, and Capt. Joseph Shoham.

CHAPTER 8

King and Sgt. Charles Willen knew Slanger and offered memories from Fort Bragg and Europe. King, for example, recalled the party that the Second Platoon had after finding the ducks at the abandoned farmhouse near Orglandes. Pvt. Lewis J. Marchand, Tampa, Florida, knew Slanger while she was at Camp Gordon in Georgia and offered insight on her.

I came to understand Dr. Isadore Schwartz not only through those who knew him during the war but through his son, Edward, whom I interviewed in person in Boston; Joseph Yanoff, who knew him; and an article in the *Quincy Patriot Ledger* by a doctor who said Schwartz was "supremely confident [justifiably] of his medical opinions . . . relentless in his pursuit of the best treatment for every patient under his care" and, most significantly, "spoke his mind honestly and forthrightly."

The military's blatant racism during World War II was well documented in *Liberators: Fighting on Two Fronts in World War II* by William Miles Potter and Nina Rosenblum (Orlando, Florida: Harcourt Brace Jovanovich, Publishers, 1992). Also helpful was *Double Victory: A Multicultural History of America in World War II* by Ronald T. Takaki (Boston: Little, Brown and Co., 2000).

For an understanding of Fort Bragg, I'm indebted to its present-day historian, Donna Barr Tabor, who sent me *Fort Bragg at War: The Station Complement* (Atlanta: U.S. Army, 1945).

CHAPTER 9

Items in Frances Slanger's possession were listed in her casualty file, obtained from the Department of the Army through a Freedom of Information Act.

I saw all issues of *Stars and Stripes* from July 4, 1944, when it first began printing in France, to November 22, 1944, when the paper reported the news of Frances Slanger's death.

Interestingly, the "Jewish bath" incident was among the few memories of Frances Slanger that immediately came to mind for all four of the still-living nurses from the Forty-fifth Field Hospital.

Frances's role as peacekeeper was documented by eyewitness reports and "Buddy Book" entries.

The German bomber that nearly crashed into the Forty-fifth Field Hospital was described by Pvt. William King.

SOURCE NOTES

Dr. John Bonzer told of Frances giving the German soldier the same treatment she gave to American soldiers, which was common for all the nurses in the Forty-fifth.

Joseph Shoham recalled the purchase and naming of "Penny," the Second Platoon's dog, in Paris following the city's liberation by American forces and remembered Isadore Schwartz buying and playing his trumpet.

Venereal disease reports on the Forty-fifth were gleaned from "Monthly Sanitary Reports" found among records of the unit at the National Archives.

Frances's experience of finding the soldier snuggling with his dog was from a poem she'd written about the incident, found in the Frances Slanger Collection, History of Nursing Archives, The Howard Gotlieb Archives Research Center at Boston University. Her "Diane Macy" short story is contained in the same collection.

Finally, the Sabbath services were recalled by Shoham, who helped organize them.

CHAPTER 10

The Forty-fifth Field Hospital's bloody stint in Bastogne was chronicled in the unit's annual report, found at the National Archives.

The photograph of Frances and the woman in Belgium were found in The Howard Gotlieb Archives Research Center. The photograph of her and Tiny Schwartz was discovered in a photo album belonging to Sallylou Cummings.

In a personal interview, Erich Dahmen, a hotel owner in Elsenborn, Belgium, provided insight into the place Slanger died. He was eight years old when German troops marched into town on May 10, 1940—"at 3 P.M.," he recalled. And he remembered Americans troops arriving four years later.

Cummings told, and others confirmed, the story of Sallylou's "Nazi" swimsuit unveiling. "Monty" Montague and Willen recalled the letter from Eva Slanger beckoning her daughter to come home because of her father's illness.

The March 1942 fire from which Eva Slanger and other family members narrowly escaped was well documented by an article

273

(complete with a photo of Frances's two nephews, Irwin and Jerry) in a Boston newspaper and by Frances's typewritten comments flanking the article in her chapbook.

The annual report of the 179th Medical Battalion, under which the Forty-fifth Field Hospital operated, offered details about the unit being in Elsenborn. It was found in the National Archives.

Two books by Charles Whiting were helpful in understanding the Siegfried Line, near where the Forty-fifth was camped when Frances died: *Siegfried: The Nazis' Last Stand* (Briarcliff Manor, N.Y.: Stein and Day Publishers, 1984) and *The Battle of Hürtgen Forest* (New York: Crown Publishers, 1989).

Edith Nourse Rogers's visit to Elsenborn was referred to in her personal papers, found in Schlesinger Library at the Radcliffe Institute for Advanced Study, Harvard University, Cambridge, Massachusetts. None of the the Forty-fifth nurses or doctors I interviewed recalled seeing Rogers. However, after Slanger's death, the congresswoman eulogized Frances on the House floor November 27, 1944, saying, "Lieutenant Slanger typifies the spirit of all the nurses overseas. I visited the tented evacuation hospital myself. . . ." Rogers may have misspoke when she said "evacuation" hospital because the Forty-fifth was a "field" hospital. But that she did, in fact, visit the Forty-fifth seems likely, given that, on May 27, 1945, in remarks made at a memorial for nurses at Arlington National Cemetery, she told Slanger's story and said "I saw her at the hospial. . . ."

The October 10, 1944, incident in which a U.S. reconnaissance platoon just south of Elsenborn ran into a field of "Bouncing Betties" was chronicled in Stephen Ambrose's *Citizen Soldiers*.

A newspaper published by the 134th Medical Group, under which the Forty-fifth Field Hospital operated, reported the eighteen-man German scout patrol that killed two GIs and stole their jeeps on the Forty-fifth's "front porch."

A daily Supreme Headquarters, Allied Expeditionary Force situation map of the Twelfth Army Group, obtained through the National Archives, showed where American, British, and German units were located in the Elsenborn area on October 21, 1944, the day Frances Slanger died. A report issued from the V Corps Headquarters on October 21, 1944, also offered a summary on the situation.

The *Detroit News* contained articles about Maj. Herman Lord following his death in October 1944.

CHAPTER 11

What happened in Auschwitz on the day Frances Slanger died, October 21, 1944, was known because of an incredibly detailed book, *Auschwitz Chronicle*, edited by Danuta Czech (New York: Henry Holt and Company, 1989). The Germans were meticulous at record-keeping and the *Chronicle* is horrific evidence of their methodic madness.

Specific details about the deadly attack on the Second Platoon came from a number of sources. First and foremost were those who were there: Shoham, Bonzer, Michalove, King, and Willen. (None of the nurses who were there that night are still living.) The Forty-fifth's Annual Report offers some detail, though surprisingly little, on the attack, as do the unit's Company Morning Reports. Newspaper articles written by Catherine Coyne, a war correspondent for the *Boston Herald*, and by Associated Press reporter Ruth Cowan offered additional context.

Writer David Cohn provided physical detail description of what Henri-Chapelle Cemetery was like in 1944 through a magazine article he wrote ("The Grave at Henri-Chapelle." *Tomorrow*, September 1946). Cohn visited Slanger's grave shortly after reading about her letter and death in the November 22, 1944, issue of *Stars and Stripes*.

A letter from Orlow A. Rusher, the Forty-fifth Field Hospital's chaplain, to Eva Slanger said Rabbi Sydney Lefkowitz, an army chaplain, had spoken at her service. The Frances Slanger Collection, History of Nursing Archives, The Howard Gotlieb Research Center at Boston University contains photographs of Frances's grave in Belgium, taken by an army photographer.

Finally, that it snowed on the day of her burial—the season's first snowfall on the war's Western Front—was gleaned from the next day's issue of *Stars and Stripes* (October 25, 1944).

CHAPTER 12

Frances's eldest nephew, Irwin Sidman, recalled the details of his mother and grandmother receiving the news about his aunt's death. Eight years old at the time, he was present when the Western Union messenger came to the door.

The letters from soldiers written in response to Frances's editorial in *Stars and Stripes* are held at the National Archives. Only one of the letters, Pvt. Millard Ireland's, was actually printed in the newspaper, though *Stars and Stripes* said that hundreds had been received.

Eva Slanger saved dozens and dozens of newspaper clippings about Frances that were sent to her from cities and towns across the United States. These, along with Frances's Purple Heart, wound up in the Frances Slanger Collection, History of Nursing Archives, The Howard Gotlieb Archival Research Center at Boston University.

Other information at Boston University regarding Frances's death included the letter from Louise Ostermann of Liège, Belgium, involving the upkeep of Frances's grave; the article by soldier "Spec" McClure, former colleague of Hollywood gossip columnist Hedda Hopper; and a complete transcript of WABC's "We the People" radio program featuring Frances.

Details of the Russian soldiers finding the last remaining Jews in the Lødz Ghetto on January 19, 1945, were from a journal entry by Jakub Pozanski in *Lodz Ghetto: Inside a Community Under Siege*, edited by Alan Adelson and Robert Lapides (New York: Viking, 1989).

A copy of the Memorial Day 1945 speech by Charles Sawyer, the U.S. ambassador to Belgium, was uncovered at the National Archives. The Harry S. Truman Library in Independence, Mo., provided photos of Sawyer.

The launching of a ship was detailed wonderfully in John H. La Dage's *Merchant Ships: A Pictorial Study* (Cambridge, Maryland: Cornell Maritime Press, 1955).

SOURCE NOTES

Most of the detail about the *Frances Y. Slanger* hospital ship came from Pvt. Wesley R. Knuth, an army medic on the ship, and from Emory Massman's *Hospital Ships of World War II* (Jefferson, North Carolina: McFarland & Company, Inc., Publishers, 1999).

A copy of the official order from Gen. George C. Marshall, the U.S. Army Chief of Staff, designating the *Saturnia* as the new hospital ship *Frances Y. Slanger* was found at the National Archives.

EPILOGUE

Details of the 6,248 war dead coming home—some papers reported the number at 5,600—and Frances Slanger's casket being chosen to symbolically honor her comrades were found in a number of newspaper articles based on Associated Press and International News Service reports. One paper reported that Slanger's casket was chosen at random. That's possible, but given that hers was the lone female body aboard the ship, it's a coincidence almost too great to believe.

AFTERWORD

The bulk of this chapter is based on information gleaned from my visit to France and Belgium from September 9, 2001, to September 18, 2001.

BIBLIOGRAPHY

Aaron, Freida. *Bearing the Unbearable: Yiddish and Polish Poetry in the Ghettos and Concentration Camps.* Albany, N.Y.: State University of New York Press, 1990.

Adelson, Alan, and Robert Lapides. *Lodz Ghetto: Inside a Community Under Siege.* New York: Viking, 1989.

Allen, Frederick Lewis. *Only Yesterday: An Informal History of the 1920's.* New York: Harper & Row, 1931.

Allison, Alida. *Isaac Bashevis Singer: Children's Stories and Childhood Memoirs.* New York: Twayne Publishers, 1996.

Ambrose, Stephen E. *Band of Brothers.* New York: Touchstone, 1992.

———. *Citizen Soldiers.* New York: Touchstone, 1997.

———. *D-Day.* New York: Touchstone, 1994.

Army Life. Washington, D.C.: War Department, 1944.

Arnold, Stanislaw, and Mariann Zychows. *Outline History of Poland.* Warsaw: Polonia Publishing House, 1962.

Articles of War: The Spectator Book of World War II. London: Grafton Books, 1989.

Astor, Gerald. *The Greatest War: Volume II.* New York: Warner Books, 1999.

Balkoski, Joseph. *Beyond the Beachhead: The 29th Infantry Division in Normandy.* Mechanicsburg, Pa.: Stackpole Books, 1989.

Banner, Lois W. *Women in Modern America.* New York: Harcourt Brace Jovanovich, Inc., 1974.

Baum, Charlotte, Paula Hyman, and Sonya Michel. *The Jewish Woman in America.* New York: Plume, 1975.

Benson, Evelyn. *As We See Ourselves: Jewish Women in Nursing.* Indianapolis, Ind.: Sigma Theta Tau International Honor Society of Nursing, 2001.

Bendersky, Joseph W. *The "Jewish Threat."* New York: Basic
   Books, 2000.
Bluejackets' Manual. Annapolis, Md.: United States Naval Institute,
   1943.
Boody, Bertha M. *A Psychological Study of Immigrant Children at
   Ellis Island.* Baltimore: The Williams & Wilkins Company,
   1926.
Bridgman, Jon. *The End of the Holocaust: The Liberation of the
   Camps.* Portland, Ore.: Areopagitica Press, 1990.
Brownstone, David M., Douglass L. Brownstone, and Irene M.
   Franck. *Island of Hope, Island of Tears.* New York: Rawson,
   Wade Publishers, Inc., 1979.
Carpenter, Iris. *No Woman's World.* Cambridge: The Riverside
   Press, 1946.
Chyet, Stanley F. *Lives and Voices: A Collection of American Jewish
   Memoirs.* Philadelphia: The Jewish Publication Society of
   America, 1972.
Cohen, Rose. *Out of the Shadow.* Ithaca, N.Y.: Cornell University
   Press, 1995.
Cohen, Sandor, ed. *Women in the Military: A Jewish Perspective.*
   Washington, D.C.: The National Museum of American
   Jewish Military History, 1999.
Collins, Lawrence D. *56th Evac Hospital: Letters of a WWII Army
   Doctor.* Waco, Texas: University of North Texas Press, 1995.
Cooper, Leo. *At the Eleventh Hour.* Barnsley, South Yorkshire: Pen
   & Sword Ltd., 1998.
Costello, John. *Virtue Under Fire: How World War II Changed Our
   Social and Sexual Attitudes.* Boston: Little, Brown and
   Company, 1985.
Courtney, Richard D. *Normandy to Bulge.* Carbondale, Ill.:
   Southern Illinois Press, 1997.
Cowdrey, Albert E. *Fighting for Life.* New York: The Free Press,
   1994.
Cox, Deborah R., and Carolyn M. Feller, eds. *Highlights in the
   History of the Army Nurse Corps.* Washington, D.C.: U.S.
   Army Center of Military History, 2001.

Currey, Cecil B. *Follow Me and Die*. Briarcliff Manor, N.Y.: Stein and Day Publishers, 1984.

Czech, Danuta, ed. *Auschwitz Chronicle*. New York: Henry Holt and Company, 1989.

Daniels, Roger. *Coming to America: A History of Immigration and Ethnicity in American Life*. New York: HarperCollins Publishers, 1990.

Davis, Cortney, and Judy Schaefer, eds. *Between the Heartbeats*. Iowa City, Iowa: University of Iowa Press, 1995.

Diner, Hasia R. *In the Almost Promised Land*. Westport, Conn.: Greenwood Press, 1977.

Dobroszycki, Lucjan. *Survivors of the Holocaust in Poland*. New York: M. E. Sharpe, Inc., 1994.

Dobroszycki, Lucjan, ed. *The Chronicle of the Lodz Ghetto 1941–1944*. Yale, Conn.: Yale University Press, 1984.

Dwork, Deborah, and Robert Jan van Pelt. *Auschwitz, 1270 to the Present*. New York: W. W. Norton & Company, Inc., 1996.

Eckener, Hugo. *My Zeppelins*. New York: Arno Press, 1980.

Elphick, Peter. *Liberty: The Ships That Won the War*. Annapolis, Md.: Naval Institute Press, 2001.

Fessler, Diane Burke. *No Time for Fear: Voices of American Military Nurses in World War II*. East Lansing, Mich.: Michigan State University Press, 1996.

Fort Bragg at War: The Station Complement. Atlanta: U.S. Army, 1945.

Framer, Sarah. *Martyred Village*. Berkeley, Calif.: University of California Press, 1999.

Frank, Anne. *The Diary of a Young Girl*. New York: Pocket Books, 1952.

Friedman-Kasaba, Kathie. *Memories of Migration*. Albany, N.Y.: State University of New York Press, 1996.

Ganter, Raymond. *Roll Me Over*. New York: Ballantine, 1997.

Gawne, Jonathan. *Spearheading D-Day*. Paris: Histoire & Collections, 1999.

Gilbert, Martin. *A History of the Twentieth Century*. New York: HarperCollins, 1998.

——. *The First World War.* New York: Henry Holt and Company, Inc., 1994.

——. *Jewish History Atlas.* London: Weidenfeld and Nicolson, 1969.

Glickman, William. *In the Mirror of Literature.* New York: Living Books, Inc., 1966.

Goodhart, Arthur. *Poland and the Minority Races.* New York: Arno Press & The New York Times, 1971.

Goodwin, Dorothy Kearns. *No Ordinary Time.* New York: Touchstone, 1994.

Hall, Tony, ed. *D-Day: Operation Overlord.* New York: Smithmark Publishers Inc., 1993.

Hebras, Robert. *Oradour-sur-Glane: The Tragedy Hour by Hour.* Les Chemins de la Memoire et Robert Hebras, 2001.

Henderson, Aileen Kilgore. *Stateside Soldier: Life in the Women's Army Corps, 1944–1945.* Columbia, S.C.: University of South Carolina Press, 2001.

Hentoff, Nat. *Boston Boy.* New York: Alfred A. Knopf, 1986.

Hertzberg, Arthur. *The Jews in America.* New York: Columbia University Press, 1997.

Hitler, Adolf. *Mein Kampf.* New York: Reynal & Hitchcock, 1939.

Hoffman, Eva. *Shtetl: The Life and Death of a Small Town and the World of Polish Jews.* Boston: Houghton Mifflin Company, 1997.

Holm, Jeanne. *Women in the Military: An Unfinished Revolution.* Novato, Calif.: Presidio Press, 1982.

The Holocaust Chronicle. Lincoln, Ill: Publications International, Ltd., 2001.

Hoyt, Edwin P. *The G.I.'s War.* New York: Cooper Square Press, 2000.

Jackson, Kathi. *They Call Them Angels: American Military Nurses of World War II.* Westport, Conn.: Praeger Publishers, 2000.

Johnson, Paul. *A History of the American People.* New York: HarperCollins, 1997.

——. *A History of the Jews.* New York: Harper & Row, 1987.

Jones, James. *WWII.* New York: Ballantine, 1975.

Katz, Alfred. *Poland's Ghettos at War*. New York: Twayne Publishers, Inc., 1970.

Kleinberg, S. J. *Women in the United States, 1830–1945*. New Brunswick, N.J.: Rutgers University Press, 1999.

Krause, Jens. *War for an Afternoon*. New York: Random House, 1968.

Kuhn, Betsy. *Angels of Mercy*. New York: Atheneum, 1999.

La Dage, John H. *Merchant Ships: A Pictorial Study*. Cambridge, Md.: Cornell Maritime Press, 1955.

Landman, Isaac, ed. *The Universal Jewish Encyclopedia*. New York: The Universal Jewish Encyclopedia, Inc., 1942.

Lanker, Brian, and Nicole Newnham. *They Drew Fire: Combat Artists of World War II*. New York: TV Books, 2000.

Levine, Hillel, and Lawrence Harmon. *The Death of an American Jewish Community: A Tragedy of Good Intentions*. New York: The Free Press, 1992.

Levinson, David, and Melvin Embers. *American Immigrant Cultures: Builders of a Nation*. New York: Simon & Schuster Macmillan, 1997.

Lewis, Jon E., ed. *Eye-Witness D-Day*. New York: Carroll & Graf Publishers, Inc., 1994.

Linderman, Gerald. F. *The World Within War*. New York: The Free Press, 1997.

Lookstein, Haskel. *Were We Our Brothers' Keepers? The Public Response of American Jews to the Holocaust, 1938–1944*. New York, N.Y.: Hartmore House, 1985.

MacDonald, Charles B. *The Siegfried Line Campaign*. Washington, D.C.: Office of the Chief of Military History, Department of the Army, 1963.

Marcus, Joseph. *Social and Political History of the Jews in Poland, 1919–1939*. Berlin: Mouton Publishers, 1983.

Martin, Ralph. *The G.I. War*. New York: Little, Brown & Company, 1967.

Masfrand, Pierre, and Guy Pauchou. *Oradour-sur-Glane: A Vision of Horror*. National Association of the Families of the Martyrs of Oradour-sur-Glane, 1997.

Massman, Emory A. *Hospital Ships of World War II.* Jefferson,
N.C.: McFarland & Company, Inc., Publishers, 1999.

Mauldin, Bill. *Up Front.* New York: Award Books, 1976.

McEntee, Girard Lindsley. *Military History of the World War.* New
York: Charles Scribner's Sons, 1937.

Medical Department Units of a Theater of Operations. Washington,
D.C.: War Department, 1945.

Medical Field Manual. Washington, D.C.: War Department, 1941.

Medical Soldier's Handbook. Harrisburg, Pa.: The Military Service
Publishing Co., 1942.

Meyer, Robert Jr. *The Stars and Stripes Story of World War II.* New
York: David McKay Company, Inc., 1960.

Mindel, Charles H., and Robert W. Habenstein. *Ethnic Families in
America.* New York: Elsevier, 1976.

Morse, Arthur D. *While Six Million Died.* New York: Random
House, 1967.

National Polish Committee of America. *The Jews in Poland:
Official Reports of The American and British Investigating
Missions.* Chicago: The National Polish Committee of
America, 1920.

Niezabitowska, Malgorzata. *Remnants: The Last Jews of Poland.*
New York: Friendly Press, Inc., 1986.

Norman, Elizabeth M. *We Band of Angels: The Untold Story of
American Nurses Trapped on Bataan by the Japanese.* New York:
Pocket Books, 1999.

Novotny, Ann. *Strangers at the Door.* New York: Bantam Books,
1972.

O'Connor, Thomas H. *Boston A to Z.* Cambridge, Mass.: Harvard
University Press, 2000.

The Officer's Guide. Harrisburg, Pa.: The Military Service
Publishing Co., 1943.

Paludeine, David Sean. *Land of the Free: A Journey to the American
Dream.* New York: Gramercy Books, 1998.

Pearson, Carol S. *Awakening the Heroes Within.* San Francisco:
HarperSanFrancisco, 1991.

Petillo, Carol. *Douglas MacArthur: The Philippine Years.*

Bloomington, Indiana: Indiana University Press, 1981.

Pitkin, Thomas M. *Keepers of the Gate: A History of Ellis Island.* New York: New York University Press, 1975.

Potter, William Miles, and Nina Rosenblum. *Liberators: Fighting on Two Fronts in World War II.* Orlando, Fla.: Harcourt Brace Jovanovich, Publishers, 1992.

Poulos, Paula Nassen. *A Woman's War Too: U.S. Women in the Military in World War II.* Washington, D.C.: National Archives and Records Administration, 1996.

Reporting World War II: American Journalism 1938–1946. New York: The Library of America, 1995.

Reporting World War II: Part Two, American Journalism 1944–1946. New York: The Library of America, 1995.

Rooney, Andy. *My War.* New York: Times Books, 1995.

Rosenfarb, Chava. *Of Lodz and Love.* Syracuse, N.Y.: Syracuse University Press, 2000.

Russell, Francis. *The Great Interlude: Neglected Events and Persons from the First World War to the Depression.* New York: McGraw-Hill Book Company, 1964.

Ryan, Cornelius. *The Longest Day.* New York: Simon and Schuster, Inc., 1959.

Sammarco, Anthony Mitchell. *Boston's South End.* Charleston, S.C.: Arcadia Publishing, 1998.

Sarna, Jonathan D., and Ellen Smith. *The Jews of Boston.* Boston: The Combined Jewish Philanthropies of Greater Boston, Inc., 1995.

Sarnecky, Mary T. *A History of the U.S. Army Nurse Corps.* Philadelphia: University of Pennsylvania Press, 1999.

Seeley, Charlotte Palmer, comp. *American Women and the U.S. Armed Forces.* Washington, D.C.: National Archives and Records Administration, 2000.

Sewell, Patricia W., ed. *Healers in World War II: Oral Histories of Medical Corps Personnel.* Jefferson, N.C.: McFarland & Company, Inc., 2001.

Sforza, Eula Awbrey. *A Nurse Remembers.* Batavia, Ill.: Parkway Press, Inc., 1991.

Shilleto, Carl, and Mike Tolhurst. *D-Day and the Battle for Normandy.* New York: Interlink Books, 2000.

Shirer, William L. *The Rise and Fall of the Third Reich.* New York: Crest Books, 1956.

Sierakowiak, Dawid. *The Diary of Dawid Sierakowiak: Five Notebooks from the Lodz Ghetto.* New York: Oxford University Press, 1996.

Singer, I. J. *The Brothers Ashkenazi.* London: Allison & Busby, 1980.

Smith, William Carlson. *Americans in the Making: The Natural History of the Assimilation of Immigrants.* New York: D. Appleton-Century Company, 1939.

Sorel, Nancy Caldwell. *The Women Who Wrote the War.* New York: Perennial, 1999.

Swift, Michael, and Michael Sharpe. *Historical Maps of World War II Europe.* London: PRC Publishing Ltd., 2000.

Syrop, Konrad. *Poland: Between the Hammer and the Anvil.* London: Robert Hale, 1968.

Takaki, Ronald T. *Double Victory: A Multicultural History of America in World War II.* Boston: Little, Brown and Co., 2000.

Terkel, Studs. *The Good War.* New York: Pantheon Books, 1984.

Tomblin, Barbara Brooks. *G.I. Nightingales: The Army Nurse Corps in World War II.* Lexington, Kentucky: The University Press of Kentucky, 1996.

Trout, Charles H. Boston, *The Great Depression and the New Deal.* New York: Oxford University Press, 1977.

Tuchman, Barbara. *The Guns of August.* New York: Dell, 1962.

Tuszynska, Agata. *Lost Landscapes: In Search of Isaac Bashevis Singer and the Jews of Poland.* New York: William Morrow and Company, Inc., 1998.

Vaught, Willma L. *The Day America Said "Thanks."* Washington, D.C.: Women's Military Press, 1999.

Vishniac, Roman. *Polish Jews.* New York: Schocken Books, 1965.

White, Theodore H. *In Search of History: A Personal Adventure.* New York: Warner Books, 1978.

Whiting, Charles. *The Battle of Hürtgen Forest.* New York: Crown Publishers, 1989.

———. *Siegfried: The Nazis' Last Stand.* Briarcliff Manor, N.Y.: Stein and Day Publishers, 1984.

Williams, Mary H. *United States Army in World War II.* Washington, D.C.: Center of Military History, 1994.

Wright, Mike. *What They Didn't Tell You about World War II.* Novato, Calif: Presidio Press, 1998.

Wyman, David S. *The Abandonment of the Jews: America and the Holocaust, 1941–1945.* New York: The New Press, 1984.

ACKNOWLEDGMENTS

Writing a book is a little like operating a field hospital: Success depends on dozens of people, all of whom play different roles but are linked by one thing: their willingness to make extraordinary sacrifices for others. In this case, for me. And I'm deeply indebted to them.

Nathan Fendrich discovered the letter written by Frances Slanger and believed so passionately in her words that he convinced me to write a newspaper column about her.

Dr. John Bonzer and Sallylou Cummings Bonzer read that column and, as part of the same Forty-fifth Field Hospital Unit as Frances, shared their memories, scrapbooks, time, and home with me, time and again, over a two-year period.

On my twentieth "cold call," I connected with Beverly and Stanley Sidman of Plymouth, Mass., distant relatives of Frances Slanger's who were able to put me in touch with one of her three nephews, Irwin Sidman, who knew the woman better than anyone else alive.

Sidman, the oldest of three nephews, patiently put up with waves of email questions—and twice welcomed me to Boston for interviews. Frances's other two nephews, James Sidman of Attleboro, Mass., and Francis Sidman of Lakeland, Fla., shared what they know about their aunt.

Joseph Shoham of Reston, Va., a captain in the Forty-fifth, was a fount of knowledge about the hospital unit, and his wife, Ethel, a most gracious host on my two visits.

Dr. John Greenwood, chief, Office of Medical History, Office of the Surgeon General, U.S. Army, constantly went the extra mile in furnishing me with information from his office in Falls Church, Va.

Emory Massman, whose book, *Hospital Ships of World War II*,

ACKNOWLEDGMENTS

included a chapter on the *Frances Y. Slanger*, pointed me to archives at Boston University that proved to be the "mother lode" of Slanger information.

When I discovered myself stymied at the National Archives, researcher Richard Boylan dropped what he was doing and took me deep into the basement caverns to find a Frances Slanger file that included dozens of letters from GIs responding to her *Stars and Stripes* letter.

Frances's childhood friend, Milton Zola, the lone person to respond to classified ads I had published in the *Boston Globe*, not only shared memories of Frances and her fruit-peddler father, but gave me a personal tour through the South End and Roxbury areas where she grew up.

My agent, Ted Weinstein, took the risk of casting his lot with an obscure, haggard author who'd arrived at that first meeting having been up literally all night because of printer problems. And constantly supported me through the publishing process.

My editor, Brenda Copeland, emerged as the rarest of editors, one who performed major surgery when necessary, offered major encouragement when necessary, and, despite the long journey, never lost her zany sense of humor.

To all these people I offer heartfelt thanks.

However, I reserve my utmost appreciation for a research assistant without whom this book would have been impossible to write. After hearing about my project, Pat Gariepy volunteered to join "Team Slanger" with gusto. With a passion for military history and a gumshoe's instincts, he looked under rocks I didn't even know existed. He refused to quit. And, best of all, he believed in the Frances Slanger story—and in me. I am forever grateful to him.

Beyond Pat Gariepy and Brenda Copeland, nobody did as much editing as Ann Petersen and Molly Petersen, whose imprint of excellence is found throughout the book. My sister, novelist Linda Crew, not only edited my original draft but offered an abundance of advice that proved invaluable. Jane Kirkpatrick, friend and novelist, edited the book and suggested a key structural change—and, in so doing, blew on the embers of a dying book. Others who

---

helped improve the story were Carrie Petersen, Dan Roberts, Karlann Greenwood, and Nancy Shattuck-Smallwood.

World War II enthusiast Ron Palmer read rough drafts, loaned me books, interviewed sources while in Europe, and was a constant source of encouragement.

Beyond Sallylou Cummings Bonzer, I thank the other nurses of the Forty-fifth who granted me personal interviews—and allowed many phone and letter follow-ups: Betty Belanger Quinn, Manchester, N.H.; Mae "Monty" Montague Bowen, Dover, Del.; and Dorothy Richter Lewis, Rehoboth Beach, Del.

I thank Jim Michalove and honor the memory of his father, Capt. Fred Michalove, who, at his assisted-living home in Rhode Island, shared his experiences with me. I'm only sorry "Mike," who died the year after I interviewed him, never got to see the book.

A tip of the helmet goes to soldiers who offered insight about Frances and the Forty-fifth: William King, Lewis J. Marchand, Charles Willen, and Emanuel Berson. Wesley Knuth, a medic aboard the *Frances Y. Slanger*, shared about the ship.

Edward Schwartz, son of Dr. Isadore Schwartz, met with me in Boston about his father and helped me better understand the man. Other relatives of those in the Forty-fifth who added insight include: Kathy Rushford and Maureen Conn, daughters of 2d Lt. Christine Cox, and Scott Levick, a son of Cox; Penny Grossman, daughter of Dr. Isadore Schwartz; Thomas Knipstein, son of Pvt. Edward Knipstein; Bob and Linda Bookhammer, son and daughter-in-law of 2d Lt. Margaret Fielden; and Frances Nicoletta, niece of 2d Lt. Margaret Bowler.

Among those who added pieces to the Frances Slanger puzzle through interviews were her cousin, Sylvia Fine, and Sylvia's late husband Joseph; close Slanger family friend Joseph Yanoff and his nephew, Stuart "Skip" Yanoff; a nursing classmate of Frances's, Hazelle Ferguson; and Frances's soda shop pal, Nathan Freidman. Others include Sylvia Sokol, the first commander of Frances Y. Slanger Post No. 313; Charlotte Lieberman, a former commander of the post; and Boston City Hospital School of Nursing alums Annetta Romano, Kathryn Webster, and Dorothy Dunphy.

ACKNOWLEDGMENTS

A number of friends provided constant encouragement during this three-year project, in particular Paul Neville, Tom Penix, Jeff Wright, Mike Yorkey, and Karen Zacharias, who listened to Frances Slanger play-by-play—or at least acted like they did—on a regular basis. Others who offered support were Steve Hill, Michael Stewart, John Mills, Gordon Ruddick, and Jason and Ann Schar. Encouragement from afar came from Jeff Bradshaw, Dan Howe, Tony Campolo, and Charles Swindoll.

Marolyn Tarrant provided the undying faith of a mother and details about life for young American women during the war years.

With utter professionalism, Alex Rankin, assistant director for manuscripts at The Howard Gotlieb Archival Research Center at Boston University, hunted down an array of files on Frances and on Boston City Hospital's School of Nursing that proved invaluable.

Judith Bellafaire, chief historian of the Women in Military Service for America Memorial Foundation in Washington, D.C., was a huge help in attempting to find Forty-fifth nurses who might still be alive.

Dick Foth, Falls Church, Va., set up a meeting with Ret. Lt. Gen. Claud "Mick" Kicklighter, assistant Secretary for the Office of Policy & Planning in the Department of Veterans Affairs in Washington, D.C. Kicklighter and staff members Eileen Chandler and Lucrecia McClenney helped find key information for me.

U.S. Congressman Peter DeFazio, a Democrat from Oregon, and assistant Frank VanCleave ran interference to see that a Freedom of Information request was acted upon.

Shirley Rotbein Flaum, an expert on Jewish genealogy of people from the Lødz, Poland, area, helped construct a Slanger family tree with an assist from Petje Schröder of Lødz, a professional researcher. Harold and Bonnie Youngberg also offered genealogical guidance, as did Rabbi Asher Bar-Zev, Reeva Kimble, and the Eugene (Oregon) Jewish Genealogy Study Group. William Hoffman, author of *Polish Surnames: Origins & Meanings*, offered personal insight regarding the Slanger name itself.

Grief counselor Debra Alexander, author of *Children Changed by Trauma*, analyzed Frances's writing and helped me understand how the nurse's dark childhood might have effected the adult she became. Leah Garfield offered insight on the relationship between Jewish mothers and daughters. Dr. Glenn Petersen answered numerous medical questions.

John Miller and Peter Breaden furnished me with important books. Britni Jones and Donna Long translated French, and Brigitte Cross translated German.

In Israel, Rivka (Rikki) Freudenstein, of Jerusalem, helped translate Yiddish, with help from Abe Carrey and Norman Rosenman, both of Far Rockaway, N.Y. Oxana Korol, a staffer at Yad Vashem's Hall of Names in Jerusalem, researched "Slangers" and "Schlangers" who died in the Holocaust.

In Europe, the staff at the Utah Beach Landing Museum showed me where the Forty-fifth Field Hospital Unit most likely came ashore. Erich Dahmen shared extensively of his World War II memories of Elsenborn, Belgium, where Frances was killed. Caroline Oliver, a guide associate, and Gerald V. Arseneault, superintendent, at the Henri-Chapelle American Cemetery and Memorial in Belgium, provided valuable information. Carl and Kim Davaz offered beyond-the-call-of-duty advice as I prepped for the trip to France and Belgium.

I thank my former editor at *The Register-Guard* newspaper, Margaret Haberman, for her patience and flexibility as I juggled column- and book-writing responsibilities. The paper's librarian, Sue Boyd, made occasional informational forays on my behalf. Others at the paper who lent their support were Kevin Miller, Jim Godbold, Tina Ellis, John Heasly, and Susan Honthumb.

Author and newspaper editor Mike Thoele saved me considerable time by showing me how to index gobs of information in a data base.

Evelyn Benson, a former nurse and author of *As We See Ourselves: Jewish Women in Nursing*, was a tremendous help, as was Mary Sarnecky, author of *A History of the U.S. Army Nurse Corps*.

Other people who supplied me with information include: Jack Berman, national commander, Jewish War Veterans of the U.S.A., Washington, D.C.; Debra Cox and Maj. Jennifer Petersen, historians, Army Nurse Corps, Falls Church, Va.; Pamela Felton, former curator, Neil Goldman, past president, Florence Levine, head of the women's collection, and Tom Wildenberg and Jon West-Bey, archivists, the National Museum of American Jewish Military History, Washington, D.C.; Donna Barr Tabor, Fort Bragg (N.C.) Historian; and Bob Tarrant of Corvallis, Ore., a former Navy officer whose ship was positioned off Normandy Beach at the same time the *Pendleton* was.

Archivists and museum curators I'm indebted to include: Loretta Ashford, National Personnel Records Center in St. Louis, Mo.; Mary Beth Dunhouse, Boston Public Library; Ned Hammond, The American Merchant Marine Museum, Kings Point, N.Y.; the Steamship Historical Society, Baltimore, Md.; Eleanor Kelley, Boston Public Schools; Thomas M. Jones, Department of the Army, Alexandria, Va.; Charlene Neuwiller, *Stars and Stripes* newspaper, Washington, D.C.; Melissa Salazar, New Mexico State Records Center and Archives, Santa Fe, N.M.; Kristen Swett, City of Boston; Ellen M. Shea, Schlesinger Library at the Radcliffe Institute for Advanced Study, Harvard University, Cambridge, Mass.; and Pauline Testerman, Harry S. Truman Library, Independence, Mo.

Librarians who added pieces to the puzzle include: Barbara Jenkins and Katie Sloan, University of Oregon's Knight Library in Eugene, Ore.; Mary McGown-Pettibone and Jim Gallagher, Beebe Library, Boston University; Suzanne Nichelson, Beverly (Mass.) Public Library; Aaron Schmidt and Henry Scannell, Boston Public Library; Ann Tumavicus and Joan Ackerman, the Westfield (Mass.) Athenaeum; Laurie Vanasse, the *Springfield* (Mass.) *Union-News*; and the library staff at the *Detroit News*.

Thanks, also, to: Ellen Berlin, director of corporate communications, Boston Medical Center; Don Burton and Tricia Noonan, the *Boston Herald*; Ramona Caplan, Albuquerque, N.M.; Clare Donaher, Washington, D.C.; Mary Gunn, counselor, Department of Veterans Affairs, Eugene, Ore.; Evelyn Noakes Hadaway, a former WWII army nurse, Bellevue, Wash.; Kara Honthumb-Lange, Boston; Peggy Engel, Bethesda, Md.; State Rep. Joe Manning,

Boston, Mass.; Scott McKee, Eugene Police Department, Eugene, Ore.; Andy Nelson, photographer, the *Christian Science Monitor*, Washington, D.C.; Brent Northup, professor, Carroll College in Helena, Mont.; Bob Stewart, veterinarian, Eugene, Ore.; Joanne Tierney, aide to Rep. William Galvin, State House, Boston, Mass.; and Scott Troppy, Boston University alumni office.

I thank my son Ryan, my daughter-in-law Susan, and my son Jason for their faith and encouragement. And I thank my wife, Sally Jean, who not only deftly walked that tightrope of being author's editor and spouse, but when I was ready to quit, wouldn't let me.

Finally, I honor my late father, Warren, a navy landing-craft coxswain during World War II, and all who served in medical units during this tumultuous time. The sacrifices of these unsung heroes helped win a war, restored freedom to the world, and reflected honorably the spirit of their fellow soldier, Frances Slanger.

To contact the author: www.bobwelch.net

INDEX

INDEX

INDEX

Hunter, Kent, 227
Hürtgen Forest, Battle of the, 179, 252
Hussein, Saddam, 248
Hynes, John B., 239
Hyvernaud family, 76-77

immigration: Americans' views about, 27-28, 110; of Slanger, 10, 27-34, 110. *See also* Ellis Island; *specific person*
"In Flanders Fields" (McCrae), 55
Independent Pride of Boston (Jewish cemetery), 239
Ireland, Millard, 219-20
Israel, 243

Jackson, "Utah," 145-46
Japan, 237
"Jewish baths" comment, 159
Jewish Memorial Hospital (Boston, Massachusetts), 237, 245
Jewish War Veterans, 227
Jews: and beginning of World War II, 97-99; in Boston, 51, 52-53, 58, 66, 88, 227; in Czechoslovakia, 119, 232-33; death camps for, 116, 169, 180-81, 201, 231, 232, 233; as doctors and nurses, 81; "final solution" for, 111, 114-15; immigration of, 29; media reports about atrocities against, 116; in Poland, 13-14, 16-18, 94, 97-99, 114, 115-16, 117, 230, 243; protests about atrocities against, 119; Slanger's concern about, 114, 117; in Slovakia, 116; social class among, 52-53; suicide among, 111; in U.S. military, 9-10, 159-60. *See also anti-Semitism; specific person*

Kämpfe, Helmut, 242
Katz, Grendla, 29
Kengigsberg family, 186
King, William, 166, 172, 204, 207
Knipstein, Edward, 208
Kohn, Edward, 256-57
Kostasky, Harry, 58

Kristallnacht (Night of the Broken Glass), 97

La Jullière, France, 191
La Madeleine, France, 43
Labrie, Irene, 71
Lake Nubanusit, 54, 69
Land, Emory Scott, 5
Le Grand Chemin, France: German attacks on, 63-64, 71-72; nurses at, 61-66, 70-72; nurses' hike to, 46-49, 61
Le Ruisseau, France, 162-66, 169-70
Lefkowitz, Sydney, 215
Lemack family, 186
Leveques, Mr. and Mrs., 77
Levi, Breina, 29
Leyman, Sidney, 229
Liberty ships, 5-7, 237
Liège, Belgium, 233
Life magazine, 112, 119
Lincoln, Abraham, 5, 258
Lincoln (Abraham) Intermediate School (Boston, Massachusetts), 55, 56, 57-58, 240
Lodz, Poland: and David and Eva's relationship, 59; Ghetto in, 98-99, 110, 111, 169, 242; Jews in, 13, 16-18, 94, 98-99, 110, 111, 114, 115-16, 117, 169, 230, 243; Slanger as child in, 10, 11, 12, 14-18, 34, 44, 51, 64, 85, 139, 140, 186, 213; and Slanger's personality, 56; Soviets in, 230, 243; in World War I, 11, 14-18, 44, 64, 98-99, 140, 186; in World War II, 98-99, 110, 111, 114, 115-16, 117, 169, 230
Lord, Herman McNeill, 81, 102, 127, 133, 143, 149, 171, 182, 193, 203; death of, 213, 214, 232; and German attack on field hospital, 207, 209; personal and professional background of, 100; wounding of, 209
Lord, Wilma, 100, 171
Luxembourg, 190, 219

MacArthur, Douglas, 12, 80, 116,

INDEX

Printed in the United States
By Bookmasters